Coronary Artery Stenting: A Case-oriented Approach

a. Severe lesions in the body of an RCA SVG. By courtesy of Dr Ulrich Sigwart, Royal Brompton Hospital, London, UK.

b. Final result after stenting in patient mentioned above (a). By courtesy of Dr Ulrich Sigwart, Royal Brompton Hospital, London, UK.

c. A severe, bulkly eccentric lesion in the proximal LCx (arrow) as well as a severe bifurcation lesion involving LAD and its diagonal branch (arrowheads). By courtesy of Dr David R Ramsdale, The Cardiothoracic Centre, Liverpool, UK.

d. Repeated angiography in patient mentioned above (c) showing that the dissection in the diagonal artery had healed satisfactorily. By courtesy of Dr David R Ramsdale, The Cardiothoracic Centre, Liverpool, UK.

Coronary Artery Stenting: A Case-oriented Approach

Edited by

Nick Curzen PhD, MRCP
Manchester Heart Centre
UK

and

Martin T Rothman FRCP, FACC, FESC
The London Chest Hospital
UK

MARTIN ■ DUNITZ

© 2001 Martin Dunitz Ltd, a member of the Taylor & Francis group

First published in the United Kingdom in 2001 by
Martin Dunitz Ltd
The Livery House
7–9 Pratt Street
London NW1 0AE

Tel: +44-(0)20-7482-2202
Fax: +44-(0)20-7267-0159
E-mail: info.dunitz@tandf.co.uk
Website: http://www.dunitz.co.uk

A CIP record for this book is available from the British Library.

ISBN 1-85317-718-0

Distributed in the United States by:
Blackwell Science Inc.
Commerce Place, 350 Main Street
Malden, MA 02148, USA
Tel: 1-800-215-1000

Distributed in Canada by:
Login Brothers Book Company
324 Salteaux Crescent
Winnipeg, Manitoba R3J 3T2
Canada
Tel: 204-224-4068

Distributed in Brazil by:
Ernesto Reichmann Distribuidora de Livros, Ltda
Rua Coronel Marques 335, Tatuape 03440-000
Sao Paulo,
Brazil

$60.00

Composition by Scribe Design, Gillingham, Kent
Printed and bound in Spain by Grafos S.A.

CONTENTS

LIST OF CONTRIBUTORS

Dr. Johanna Armstrong PhD
Cardiovascular Research Group
Division of Clinical Sciences
Sheffield
England

Dr. Christopher SR Baker BSc, MB, BS, MRCP
Department of Cardiology
Barts & The London NHS Trust
London Chest Hospital
London
England

Dr. Stephan Baldus
Kerckhoff-Klinik
Bad Nauheim
Germany

Dr. Julia Baron MB, BS, MRCP
Department of Academic Cardiology
University Hospitals
Leicester
England

Dr. Antonio Bartorelli MD
Director of Catheterisation Laboratories
Centro Cardiologico
Fondazione Monzino
Instituto di Ricovero e Cura a Carattere
Scientifico
Milano
Italy

Dr. Hans Bonnier MD
Cardiologie
Catharina Ziekenhuis
Michelangelolaan 2
Eindhoven
The Netherlands

Dr. Carl Brookes MD, MRCP
Consultant Cardiologist
Royal Brompton and Harefield NHS Trust
London
England

Dr. Bernard Chevalier MD
Centre Cardiologique du Nord
Departement de Cardiologie Interventionelle
Saint Denis Cedex
France

Dr. Antonio Colombo MD
Director Cardiac Catheterisation Laboratory
Columbus Hospital
Milan
Italy
Director of Investigational Angioplasty
Lennox Hill Hospital
New York
USA

Dr. Nick Curzen BM(Hons), PhD, MRCP
Consultant Cardiologist
Manchester Heart Centre
Manchester Royal Infirmary
Manchester
England

Dr. Stephen G. Ellis MD
The Cleveland Clinic Foundation
Cleveland OH
USA

Dr. Jean Fajadet MD
Unite De Cardiologie Interventionelle
Clinique Pasteur
Toulouse Cedex
France

Dr. Peter J Fitzgerald MD
Centre for Research in Cardiovascular
Interventions
Stanford University
Stanford CA
USA

Dr. Anthony H Gershlick BSc, MB, BS, FRCP
Department of Academic Cardiology
University Hospitals
Leicester
England

Prof. Christian W Hamm MD
Director Department of Cardiology
Kerckhoff-Klinik
Bad Nauheim
Germany

Dr. Cathy Holt PhD
Cardiovascular Research Group
Division of Clinical Sciences
Sheffield
England

Dr. Samir Kapadia MD
The Cleveland Clinic Foundation
Cleveland OH
USA

Dr. William D Knopf MD, FACC
Atlanta Cardiology Group
Atlanta GA
USA

Dr. Michael Kutryk MD, PhD, FRCPC
St Michael's Hospital
Toronto
Ontario
Canada

Dr. Thierry Lefevre MD
Institut Cardiovasculaire Paris Sud
Clinique du Bois Verrieres
Antony
France

Dr. Jurgen MR Ligthart MD
Erasmus University
Heartcenter Rotterdam
Thoraxcenter, Bd 418
University Hospital Dijkzigt
GD Rotterdam
The Netherlands

Dr. Chaim Lotan MD
Director of Interventional Cardiology
Hadassah Hospital
Ein Kerem
Jerusalem
Israel

Dr. Marie-Claude Morice MD
Institut Cardiovasculaire Paris Sud
Clinique du Bois Verrieres
Antony
France

Prof. Harald Mudra MD
Krankenhaus Neuperlach 2nd Medical Department
Munich
Germany

Dr. Christopher MH Newman MA, PhD, FRCP
Cardiovascular Research Group
Division of Clinical Sciences
Sheffield
England

Dr. Seung-Jung Park MD, PhD, FACC
Chief Division of Cardiology
Director Interventional Cardiology
Cardiovascular Centre
Asian Medical Centre
Seoul
Korea

Dr. Ian M Penn MB, BS (Hons), FRACP, FRCP
Director of Interventional Cardiology
Vancouver Hospital & Health Sciences Centre
Clinical Associate Professor of Medicine
University of British Columbia
Vancouver BC
Canada

Dr. Martin T Rothman FRCP, FACC, FESC
Department of Cardiology
Barts & The London NHS Trust
The London Chest Hospital
London
England

Dr. Manel Sabaté MD
Erasmus University
Heartcenter Rotterdam
Thoraxcenter, Bd 418
University Hospital Dijkzigt
GD Rotterdam
The Netherlands

Dr. Patrick Serruys MD, PhD, FACC, FESC
Erasmus University
Heartcenter Rotterdam
Thoraxcenter, Bd 418
University Hospital Dijkzigt
GD Rotterdam
The Netherlands

Dr. Ulrich Sigwart MD, FRCP, FACC, FESC, DocHC
Consultant Cardiologist
Royal Brompton and Harefield NHS Trust
London
England

Dr. Neil Swanson MB, BS, MRCP
Department of Academic Cardiology
University Hospitals
Leicester
England

Dr. Atsushi Takagi MD
Centre for Research in Cardiovascular Interventions
Stanford University
Stanford CA
USA

Dr. Christopher J White MD
Department of Cardiology
Ochsner Heart and Vascular Institute
New Orleans LA
USA

Prof. Harvey White MD
Cardiology Department
Green Lane Hospital
Auckland
New Zealand

ACKNOWLEDGEMENTS

The Editors would like to thank Jane Hanger for her painstaking management of the process of collection of contributions and her cheerful demeanour which has kept the editors sane through the production of this book.

The images used in this book are collected from The London Chest Hospital and we are grateful to our colleagues Drs Balcon, Kelly, Layton, Mills, and Timmis for allowing us to include some of their cases.

The production of this book has been a prolonged and time-consuming activity, particularly when combined with our everyday clinical, administrative, research, teaching and other responsibilities. We therefore wish to publicly acknowledge the patience and tolerance of our wives and families who, as usual, have borne the brunt of 'the missed other opportunities'. Florence, Alex, Emma, Alison, Harvey, and Elisabeth—thank you for your continued support.

PREFACE

The practice of stent implantation has become commonplace for most interventionists, particularly for straightforward lesions. Likewise the stent is used as the universal panacea for complications, and for complex lesion subsets. This book is intended to illustrate the many situations in which stents can be used, but moreover the book is intended to illustrate the thought processes behind the decision making, the tricks employed or considered in particular situations, by a variety of experts.

The book covers a series of anatomical subsets where stents may be used. The experts consider the angiograms of these patients, supplied by the editors, and make their comments on the choice of technology, the way it was used, how it may have been used better, or why it should not have been used at all. The experts were asked to review the angiograms as if they were those of a case they were about to perform, or one they had been asked to critique. The experts were encouraged not to hold back with their comments, and you will see they have not.

This rogues' gallery of angiograms is designed to push the frontiers, or reflect where the frontiers currently are. Because the interventionists' current border territory is restenosis we have provided two contributions on this subject to introduce radiation therapy and stent coatings. These contributions take the form of essays rather than being case-based reviews. Perhaps in the future we will be able to offer angiograms on these subjects for expert comment.

Nick Curzen & Martin T Rothman

1
Discrete lesions

Discrete lesions can be the simplest that the interventional cardiologist treats. They do raise some interesting questions, however, time and again:

- What to do about the nearby side branch?
- Should the lesion be pre-dilated?
- Are some stents better for some bits of the coronary tree compared to others?
- Is the production of a stent-like angiographic result after balloon alone adequate or is it associated with an inferior outcome compared to that of a stent?
- Do some stents have higher restenosis rates?

In this chapter we introduce the format of the rest of the book and address certain general principles that recur in ever increasingly complex settings later on.

Harald Mudra provides the following introductory comments

Discrete lesions (single lesions generally under 15 mm in length), i.e. so-called BENESTENT or STRESS lesions, represent not more than 30% of the case load in most catheterization laboratories at this time. However, it is for this type of lesion in coronary arteries of >3.0 mm that we have the most valid information with regard to improved short-term and long-term outcome after coronary stent placement as compared with plain balloon angioplasty.[1,2] This has led to the common practice of most interventionists primarily to stent these lesions. This chapter will therefore discuss neither the indication for stenting discrete lesions nor potential alternatives to the strategy of provisional stenting or different ways to achieve 'optimal balloon angioplasty' or 'stent like percutaneous transluminal coronary angioplasty' (PTCA).

One of the reasons for primarily stenting this type of lesion is the ease and predictability of the intervention: the lesions do not behave differently whether they are concentric or eccentric or whether they are on the inside of the curve or the outside of the curve of a bend. To maximize the ease and predictability of the procedure the following issues are of importance:

- Anticoagulation strategy
- Balloon sizing
- Stent type and sizing
- Is this a case for direct stenting? (no pre-dilatation)
- 'Optimization' of stent deployment

Usually patients are on chronic aspirin treatment and should receive 300 mg clopidogrel whenever possible before the procedure or immediately thereafter.[3] Since discrete lesions can be treated in less than 30 minutes we, like most investigators, usually do not use more than 5000 IU of intravenous heparin (targeting an activated clotting time between 200 and 250 seconds) thus allowing also the use of abciximab if an unexpected indication arises.

Balloons and also stents are commonly utilized with a 1.0 to 1.1 : 1.0 balloon/artery ratio, using a pressure that allows full balloon expansion and ablation of the indentation caused by the lesion on the balloon. The operator must of course be aware that at high inflation pressures the balloon compliance characteristics may become important in case high pressure leads to a stretching of the balloon, and thus unintentional oversizing of the balloon with respect to the reference vessel diameter.

To achieve an optimal lumen gain most investigators use a slotted tube, corrugated ring or multicellular type of stent. Coil stents are less frequently used because of their higher recoil as well as the potential problems of tissue prolapse resulting in a smaller post-procedural lumen diameter. However, in my opinion, coil stents still have a place in cases where there is an important side branch which I wish to preserve, or where there is a requirement for maximal flexibility and conformity of the stent.

Excessive over-expansion of the balloon proximal and distal to the target lesion during pre-dilatation should be avoided because of the risk of dissection that may necessitate the deployment of a longer stent. This issue is one of the rationales for direct stenting[4] using the standard balloon/artery ratio as previously described, ideally using a device that allows an increased force application in the middle of the stent, at the centre of the lesion (the so-called 'focal balloon' concept).[5] Direct stenting may lead to a lower restenosis rate due to less vessel trauma although this is yet to be proven.

Owing to the relation between final minimal lumen diameter or residual stenosis and expected restenosis rate in this lesion type, the operator should aim to produce a perfect post-procedural angiogram (< 10% residual stenosis in vessels ≥ 3.0 mm or even a negative residual stenosis in smaller vessels). Stent expansion should be optimized by reference to the proximal reference segment diameter taking into account tapering of the vessel. The expansion of coronary stents above these angiographic criteria based on intravascular ultrasound guidance has not proved to reduce restenosis further if these angiographic criteria are met.[6]

Case 1. Discrete lesions

75-year-old woman. Non-insulin-dependent diabetes mellitus. Stable angina.

Catheter findings: Unobstructed left coronary artery; good left ventricular function; discrete right coronary artery (RCA) lesion.

Procedure: JR4 (8F) guide with sideholes; 0.014″ high torque floppy wire. 3.0 mm monorail balloon followed by Medtronic Wiktor® 3.5 mm × 15 mm to 10 atm.

Harald Mudra:

This type of B1 lesion in the mid-RCA in a vessel with a reference diameter of > 3.0 mm represents an established indication for stenting based on the data from randomized studies. In this case direct stenting could well be discussed with two points of caution. First, guiding catheter support must be predictable and good to minimize any risk of stent dislodgement from the balloon in case the stent does not cross the lesion, and likewise a stable guide catheter position is often required if there is a need to retrieve the stent back into the guide catheter. Second, major lesion calcification should be ruled out by fluoroscopy to be sure that the stent can be fully expanded. A moderate dose of intravenous heparin (around 5000 IU) and the combination of aspirin and clopidogrel are usually sufficient and allows the patient to go home the day following the implantation procedure. The lesion is easily treated via a 6F sheath and guide catheter.

Editors' note

The presence of calcification certainly seems important when planning whether to directly stent a lesion: it can be associated with difficulty of access to the appropriate deployment site as well as with full deployment.

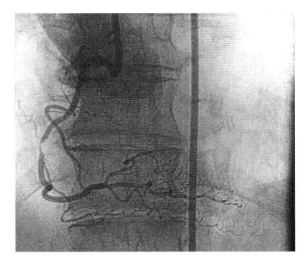

a

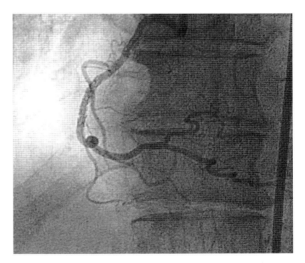

b

Figure 1.1
RCA angiogram. a) Discrete eccentric lesion in mid-RCA. b) Post-direct stent.

Case 2. Discrete lesions

70-year-old male ex-smoker. Presented with unstable angina.

Catheter findings: Good left ventricular function; Tight lesion in left anterior descending (LAD) coronary artery; remainder of coronary tree unobstructed.

Procedure: JL4 (8F) guiding catheter; 0.014″ high torque floppy wire. Lesion pre-dilated with a 3.0 mm monorail balloon, and then an ACS MULTI-LINK® 3.5 mm × 15 mm stent was deployed at 10 atm.

Harald Mudra:

This B2 lesion in the mid-LAD represents an established indication for coronary stenting with respect to restenosis reduction. Also, direct stenting could be performed based on the angiographic appearance of a relatively straight proximal LAD segment and no major lesion calcification.

Caution in some cases of this type should be paid to the patency of the medium sized first diagonal branch. In the present case the use of a protection wire placed into the diagonal artery does not seem to be necessary because there is no evidence of significant ostial disease of the diagonal. If ostial diagonal disease were seen (i.e. > 50% obstruction), pre-dilatation prior to stenting the target lesion in the LAD would be recommended because of a risk of side branch loss in about 20%.[7] If during the stenting procedure on the LAD the ostium of the diagonal side branch appears to be increasingly compromised, then a guidewire and balloon or a fixed wire balloon catheter can be placed through the stent struts to dilate the ostial side branch stenosis without causing problems for the stent in the target lesion.

The use of an ACS MULTI-LINK® stent in this case, or another stent of a comparable design, is a good option because it combines a predictable high lumen gain with easy side branch access if this becomes necessary.

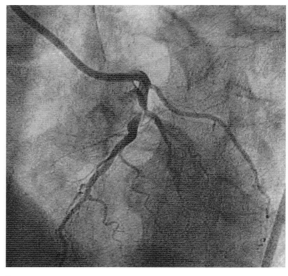

a

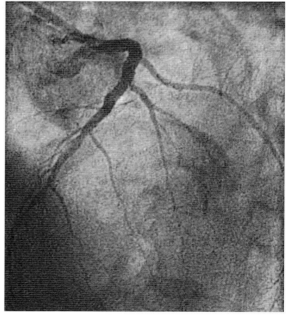

b

Figure 1.2
LCA angiogram. a) Proximal tight stenosis in LAD at 1st diagonal. b) Post-direct stent, with presentation of diagonal.

Case 3. Discrete lesions

54-year-old man. Ex-smoker. Limiting chest pain and reversible anterior ischaemia on thallium scan. Two admissions to his local hospital with angina and anterior T wave changes.

Catheter findings: Good LV; unobstructed RCA and circumflex arteries. Muscle bridge in mid-LAD.

Procedure: JL4 (8F); 0.014″ high torque floppy wire, direct stent with Cordis CrossFlex™ 3.5 mm × 25 mm to 10 atm.

Harald Mudra:

This case represents a still controversial application of coronary stenting. Stenting a muscle bridge is technically feasible but clinical benefit from this type of treatment is not proven. Late stent disruption and restenosis are reasons for caution. A muscle bridge seems to be a risk factor for the development of atherosclerosis at its proximal and distal interfaces with the normal vessel, as has been demonstrated by intravascular ultrasound.[8] For this reason, as in this case, the stents used are usually longer than in atherosclerotic stenosis and cover the adjacent normal-appearing vessel segments.

Direct stenting is usually the way to go if there are no apparent obstacles to the passage of the stent to the target segment. Some authors have described the use of stent grafts for stenting muscle bridges to reduce neointimal ingrowth. The stent graft is described in the chapter on grafts.

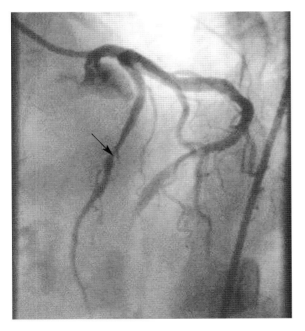
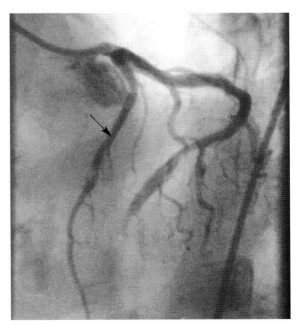

a b

Figure 1.3a–d
LCA angiogram. a) Systolic compression of mid-LAD (arrow). b) Diastolic image of LAD, no compression (arrow).

Continued

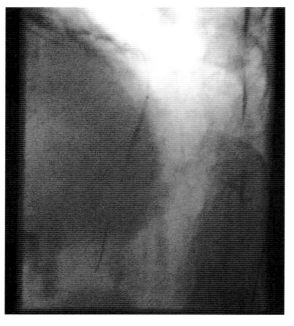

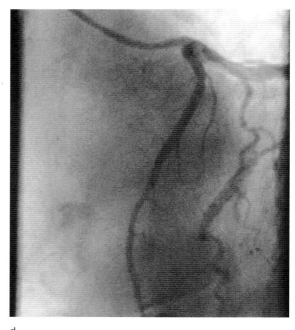

c   d

Figure 1.3 *continued*
. *c) Direct stenting, positioning of system. d) Final result after direct stenting.*

References

1. Serruys PW, Jaegere PDe, Kiemeneij F, et al. A comparison of balloon-expandable-stent implantation with balloon angioplasty in patients with coronary artery disease. N Engl J Med 1994;331:489–495.
2. Fishman DL, Leon MB, Baim DS, et al. A randomised comparison of coronary stent placement and balloon angioplasty in the treatment of coronary artery disease. N Engl J Med 1994;331:496–501.
3. Berger PB, Bell MR, Rihal CS, et al. Clopidogrel versus Ticlopidine after intracoronary stent placement. J Am Coll Cardiol 1999;34:1891–1894.
4. Figulla HR, Mudra H, Reifart N, Werner GS. Direct coronary stenting without predilatation. Cathet Cardiovasc Diagn 1998;43:245–252.

5. Mudra H, Werner F, Regar E, et al. One balloon approach for optimal Palmaz-Schatz stent implantation: The MUSCAT trial. Cathet Cardiovasc Diagn 1997;42:130–136.
6. Mudra H, Macaya C, Zahn R, et al. Interim analysis of the OPTimization with ICUS to reduce stent restenosis (OPTICUS) trial. Circulation 1998;98(Suppl. I):I–363(abstract).
7. Aliabadi D, Tilli FV, Bowers TR, et al. Incidence and angiographic predictors of side branch occlusion following high-pressure intracoronary stenting. Am J Cardiol 1997;80:994–997.
8. Ge J, Erbel R, Rupprecht HJ, et al. Comparison of intravascular ultrasound and angiography in the assessment of myocardial bridging. Circulation 1994;89:1725–1732.

2
Long segments

Long segments of disease continue to provide a technical challenge to the interventionist on a regular basis. The most frequently vexing questions in these cases can be summed up as follows:

- Which balloon length to choose?
- How much of a long area of disease should be stented?
- Should we be aiming for 'spot-stenting' of only the tightest disease?
- How much should we worry about side branches that are crossed by the stent?
- Which branches are worth 'protection'?
- Is there an ideal stent in these circumstances?
- What is the experience of the monorail Wallstent® in native vessels?
- Are there data available to suggest that abciximab is indicated solely on the grounds of 'long stented' segments?

In this chapter we present five cases covering these issues and an analysis of the way they were handled by **William D Knopf, Peter J Fitzgerald** and **Atsushi Takagi**.

William D Knopf makes these initial observations

The treatment of long diffuse disease remains problematic. Conventional percutaneous transluminal coronary angioplasty (PTCA) is associated with significant major adverse cardiac events (MACE) and restenosis rates. Although there are few randomized trials, newer techniques and technology may improve these results. There are still many controversial issues. These include:

the use of long stents or spot stents; the use of intravascular ultrasound (IVUS); the role of debulking; the treatment of side branches; and the use of IIb/IIIa inhibitors.

Conventional PTCA was routinely used for long disease. The clinical success rate, however, was only 90% with a 6% abrupt closure rate, and restenosis occurring in 55%.[1] Lesion length, vessel size, and diabetes correlated with a higher restenosis rate. Stenting has dramatically improved the acute procedural and clinical results. By contrast, the long-term results are more controversial. Although restenosis may be higher in long lesions, final minimal luminal diameter (MLD) of the stent is a strong correlate of favourable long-term results. Similarly, small vessels with long lesions have a higher restenosis rate than longer vessels > 3.0 mm.[2–4]

Stent length itself has also been associated with restenosis but this is also controversial. Proponents of spot stenting with IVUS guidance have supported lower restenosis rates in a matched study but others have felt that optimum MLD regardless of method is more important.[5,6]

Debulking seems to be important only in calcified vessels or possibly in long lesions in smaller vessels. Restenosis data using a combination of debulking and adjunctive stenting are pending. IVUS may be particularly helpful if optimal sizing or plaque morphology is in question.

IIb/IIIa inhibitors will reduce acute complications associated with coronary stenting in high risk subgroups. However, given the low rate of acute complications, these agents are used in our laboratory only for thrombus or dissection as a bailout strategy. There are little positive data to support the hypothesis that these agents contribute to a reduction in restenosis.

Case 1. Long segments

65-year-old man. High cholesterol. Presented with non-Q wave infarction and recurrent pain with anterior T wave changes.

Catheter findings: Good LV function; Long calcified tight stenosis in proximal and mid-left anterior descending (LAD); 80% proximal circumflex lesion; unobstructed dominant RCA.

Procedure: JL4 (8F); 0.014″ high torque floppy wire. Pre-dilatation with 3.0 mm monorail balloon; three overlapping stents from proximal to distal: (a) AVE GFX 3.0 mm × 40.0 mm; (b) AVE GFX 3.0 × 18.0 mm; (c) Cordis CrossFlex 3.0 mm × 15.0 mm.

William D Knopf:

The first case illustrates the treatment of a long LAD lesion with a moderately sized side branch. The lesion is calcified and the vessel tapers. Acute complications have been minimized by coronary stenting as this case demonstrates. Restenosis, however, is still a significant problem, being directly related to length of lesion, reference vessel diameter, and minimal luminal diameter (MLD) after intervention. It may also be associated with the length of the stent, but this is controversial. Because the lesion is calcified, debulking may be useful to optimize stent placement but is not mandatory and not our preference unless there is heavy calcification. Vessels of < 3.0 mm have a higher restenosis rate. Since we do not use intravascular ultrasound (IVUS), we favour covering this lesion with a long balloon-expandable stent and we would also employ post-dilatation with a 3.5 mm balloon at least proximally because this vessel tapers. We would also use a stent that allows for side branch access. Although this side branch developed a lesion after stenting, this may have been spasm and/or plaque shift. If there is no lesion at the origin initially, then nitroglycerine administration or balloon angioplasty can be performed. Usually, however, a stent is not necessary. Unless there is a significant distal dissection, we do not favour IIb/IIIa inhibitors.

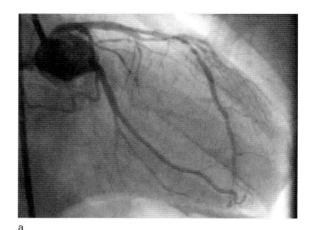

a

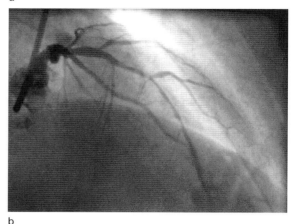

b

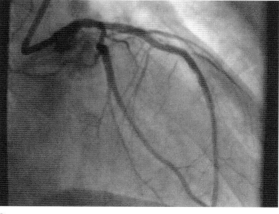

c

Figure 2.1
LCA angiogram. a) Tight mid-LAD long segment disease. b) Disease better seen in PA cronical view. c) Result after stenting.

Atsushi Takagi and
Peter J Fitzgerald:

Complete stent coverage of the majority of plaque distribution within a critical narrowing without causing tissue prolapse or dissection of atheromatous components is an important factor to maintain long-term patency following stenting. In this particular case, disease seems to begin and extend well beyond the second diagonal branch. The operator's approach to treat the extensive disease appears suitable for this particular vessel segment. In general, it is often difficult to gauge the extent of true lesion length by angiography alone.

In a separate case seen in Fig. 2.2 we demonstrate lesion length measurement by IVUS images utilizing an automated pull-back system. Distance as measured by sequential IVUS images is 8.1 mm between the LAD ostium and the first diagonal branch. An 8.0 mm stent was successfully placed within this target segment to secure sparing of the circumflex and diagonal branch.

Efficient expansion of a long stent may be restricted even by focally calcified disease in the target segment, particularly when the calcium is located in a superficial pattern. 'Softening' the lesion or increasing the radial compliance with rotational atherectomy prior to the stent placement may be an important factor for optimal stent deployment.[7] IVUS can augment the angiographic information regarding vessel morphology by providing the location and extent of calcium within the target segment.[8]

If plaque is positioned at the ostium of the branch, stenting across the orifice may cause a 'snowplough' effect of plaque, which can compromise flow into the branch. In these circumstances, branch 'jail', with slow or no flow, may be avoided by pre-dilatation of the proximal branch segment. On the angiogram of Case 1, the second diagonal branch appears 'pinched' just beyond the ostium following stenting. Two scenarios are possible: the stent may displace plaque into the branch orifice, or stent-jail may merely disturb the flow pattern into the branch by a 'honeycomb' venturi effect which yields an asymmetry of contrast filling in a patent orifice. In the first scenario, a rewiring and dilatation of the branch may be warranted. However, the latter process is benign and therefore no treatment is indicated. Again, IVUS images obtained at the bifurcation can easily distinguish plaque versus flow disturbance.[9]

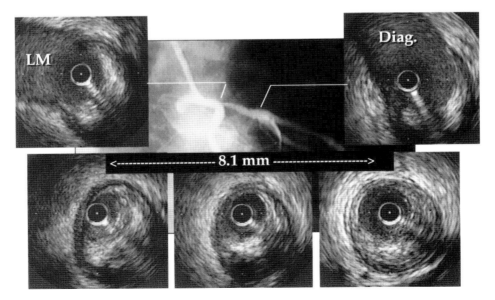

Figure 2.2
IVUS pullback. Angiogram shows extent of pullback from proximal LAD at junction of 1st diagonal, back to LM. IVUS images (clockwise): top right – at level of 1st diagonal; bottom panel – extensive plaque burden; top left: LAD/LM junction with disease in LAD ostium.

Case 2. Long segments

64-year-old man. Family history; ex-smoker. Coronary artery bypass graft (CABG) surgery 1990 (vein grafts [VGs] to left anterior descending [LAD], obtuse marginal [OM], RCA). Unstable angina with pulmonary oedema and right branch bundle block (RBBB) on ECG.

Catheter findings: Moderate LV; diffuse, mild RCA disease; proximal occlusion of LAD; long segment of disease in large circumflex. VG to OM and posterior descending artery (PDA) occluded; VG to LAD patent with good run off.

Procedure: JL4 (8F) guide; 0.014″ high torque floppy wire. Pre-dilatation with 3.0 mm monorail balloon followed by 3.5 mm × 35.0 mm ACS MULTI-LINK® stent to 12 atm.

William D Knopf:

The second case illustrates sequential lesions in the circumflex artery and raises the controversy of a long stent versus a spot stent approach. Clearly, a single stent is less costly, uses less contrast, and probably less fluoroscopy. However, it may track in the vessel with more difficulty than a short stent. On the other hand, stenting only the lesions and not the intervening normal artery will use less metal coverage and may have a better long-term result.

I would favour using two short stents to optimize both stenoses and leaving the normal artery in between. This reference vessel is approximately 3.5 mm and would suggest a favourable long-term result. If I were to use a long stent, I would ensure that my guiding catheter were coaxial. This may require a GL4 or XB4 curve rather than our standard XB3.5 or GL3.5 curve.

Atsushi Takagi and Peter J Fitzgerald:

It may be particularly important to align a stent accurately in the ostial region of the circumflex artery. An overshoot and partially 'jailing' the LAD may not be relevant to the acute clinical prognosis in the LAD. However, in the long term if the LAD subsequently becomes a target for the percutaneous approach, it may prove difficult if the circumflex stent is protruding into the LAD lumen and the metal edges of the stent may prevent delivery of interventional technology.

In case 2, the operator implanted a single stent using a double-marker balloon, which was a convenient way to determine the stent position based on angiography. 'Cine-IVUS positioning' is another helpful way to minimize the likelihood of branch jail and to cover the lesion fully. This technique is achieved by aligning the marker of the stent delivery system to the site where the IVUS transducer was placed when imaging the exit of the major branch, using the position on the frame-stored image as a reference.

When a vessel tapers quickly, it may be difficult to dilate a long stent efficiently and still scaffold the entire lesion without excessive trauma. However, a 'proper-length' single stent fitted to plaque distribution may yield the best chance for long-term success, which reduces both the cost and the chance of a vascular complication. In this situation, one may also consider a self-expandable stent, which may produce optimal, longitudinal conformation.

Previous studies have revealed higher restenosis rates with a longer stent length.[10] Stenting each individual lesion, based on IVUS image documentation, has been proposed as a 'spot stenting' technique. This is thought to be an alternative technique to sequential 'full metal jacket' stenting, expecting not only equivalent acute results but also better long-term patency. Recent studies demonstrated a lower target lesion revascularization rate following 'spot stenting' than that of traditional sequential stenting.[11] However, this issue is still controversial. Another recent study demonstrated that, once a final stent lumen is optimized, stent length becomes less predictive of subsequent target lesion revascularization.[12] Thus, IVUS may be the more efficient method to ensure the optimization of long stenting by providing cross-sectional geometric data.[13]

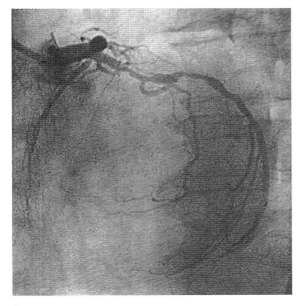

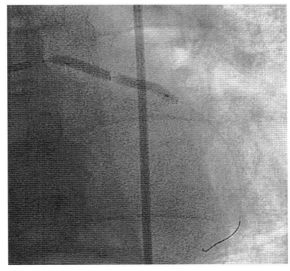

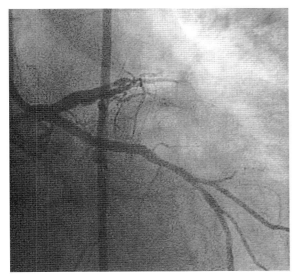

a

b

c

Figure 2.3
LCA angiogram. a) Multiple segments of disease seen in Cx. b) Stent deployment. c) Post-stenting result.

Case 3. Long segments

41-year-old man. Ex-smoker; family history. Stable, limiting angina.

Catheter findings: Good LV; unobstructed left coronary; RCA disease as shown.

Procedure: JL4 8F guide; 0.014″ High torque floppy wire. Pre-dilatation with 2.5 mm monorail balloon in several areas. Three stents overlapping from distal to proximal vessel:
(a) ACS MULTI-LINK® 3.0 mm × 25 mm; (b) Wallstent® 4.5 mm × 47 mm; (c) Wallstent® 5.0 mm × 31 mm.

William D Knopf:

This right coronary artery is a conduit vessel with few side branches until the crux where it branches into the PDA and LV branches. Because of the tight stenosis and the diffuse disease, sizing the artery is difficult. Using a small angioplasty balloon and intracoronary vasodilators, the artery size can be better assessed. If sizing is an issue, then IVUS may be helpful, especially if a self-expanding stent is used. In this case, however, the distal reference proximal to the crux appears normal. I would size my stents to this vessel. A balloon-expandable stent was chosen distally, but I would have post-dilated to 4 mm especially after seeing that a larger Wallstent® was used. Remember that the Wallstent® is sized approximately 1.0 mm greater than the reference diameter. The vessel is straightened with the Wallstent® but this is probably only a cosmetic issue and of little or no clinical significance. Since this is a conduit vessel, and side branch access is not an issue, a self-expanding stent is an acceptable choice.

Atsushi Takagi and Peter J Fitzgerald:

In treating an extremely tortuous and ectatic right coronary artery, several issues need to be considered. These include:

- Lesion length may be underestimated on angiography
- The shoulders of an angioplasty balloon often cause dissection at plaque interfaces
- The appearance of 'pseudo-stenosis' caused by a stiff guidewire may be deceiving
- The degree of shortening of self-expanding stents may be difficult to predict.

A long stent anchored into a region beyond the tortuosity may cause more uniform strain in the 'straightened' vessel. This often results in abrupt angulation at the stent edges. Fig. 2.5 below, illustrates that a 'spot stent' approach may preserve the natural curvature of the vessel.

Additionally, from a long-term consideration, restenosis may also occur in a focal pattern following this technique instead of a diffuse process that is often seen when using excessive stent lengths. The cost efficacy for treatment of diffuse restenosis in a long stent rather than focal narrowing at the edges of the spot stent approach should also be considered.

In case 3 a self-expandable stent was utilized. This stent configuration allows maximum conformity to complex anatomy with the added advantage of expansion over time. In some series, this expansion from a cross-sectional standpoint can be upward of 20% over a 6-month interval. Chronic and slow expansion resulting in a low-level force exerted from inside the artery may be preferable to direct acute balloon-forced expansion.[15]

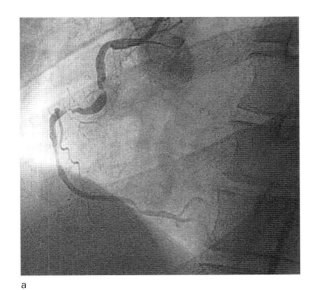

a

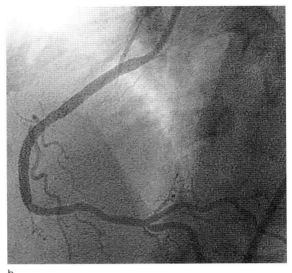

b

c

Figure 2.4
*RCA angiogram. a) Tortuous RCA with 2 discrete
lesions. b) Vessel straightened by guidewire and
stent. c) Non-contrasted image of RCA to show
extent of stent implantation.*

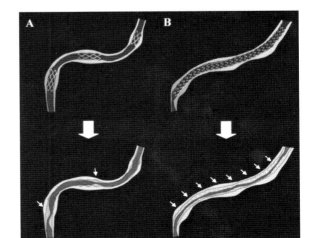

Figure 2.5
*Diagrams on left illustrate that short stents may allow
preservation of natural curvature of vessel. Right side
panel illustrates long stent placement changing shape
of vessel, this possibly leading to greater degree of
restenosis.*

Case 4. Long segments

74-year-old man. Hypertension; hypercholesterol-aemia; family history. Stable angina.

Catheter findings: Inferior hypokinesia but overall well-preserved LV; unobstructed LCA; RCA occluded.

Procedure: Amplatz Left 2 Guide; 0.014″ high torque floppy wire backed up by 1.5 mm over-the-wire balloon. Once disobliterated, pre-dilatation with 3.0 mm monorail balloon, the AVE GFX 4.0 mm × 24 mm stent across line of occlusion.

William D Knopf:

The fourth case illustrates a difficult problem as it is unclear from the history or the angiogram whether this is a chronic total occlusion or a tight lesion with collateral flow competitively filling the vessel in a retrograde fashion. A small balloon was used to pre-dilate this lesion and assess the distal artery. A single stent was used to open this lesion but I believe a shorter stent could have been used. I favour using the short-est stent necessary since restenosis has been correlated with stent length. In general an AL2 guide is reserved for high and anterior take-offs of the right coronary artery. If this is a chronic total occlusion an AL1 guide or JR4 guide may be used. Finally there is a significant distal lesion which should be stented as well, once distal flow is re-established.

Atsushi Takagi and Peter J Fitzgerald:

It is quite difficult to assess the true vessel diame-ter and true lesion length beyond the occluded zone based on the angiography. Direct stenting without pre-dilatation sometimes results in the undersizing of stent diameter and length, thus not providing proper lesion coverage. Pre-dilatation helps the operator ascertain anatomical informa-tion beyond the tight stenosis as demonstrated in this case. Instead of pre-dilatation the data of

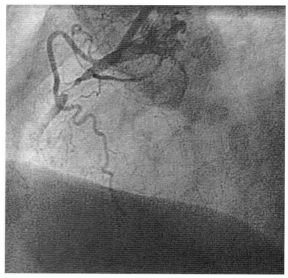

a

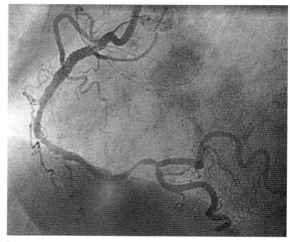

b

Figure 2.6
RCA angiogram. a) Tight proximal lesion and mid-RCA total occlusion. b) Post-stent result.

lesion length and vessel size provided by pre-intervention IVUS may guide the direct stenting properly.

Another important issue in this case was how to manage the distal stenosis which was discovered after the target stenting. Once spasm was ruled out by administrating intracoronary nitrates, three therapeutic options may be considered:

- Sequential stenting without evaluating the physiological significance of the distal stenosis

- Stenting based on the data delivered from either coronary flow reserve measurement or fractional flow reserve measurement
- Not dilating the distal stenosis and initiating an aggressive lipid-lowering programme followed by thallium scintigraphy 3 months later. As recent studies have shown, aggressive lipid-lowering therapy is highly effective in reducing the incidence of ischaemic events in patients with stable angina.

We would support the latter strategy.[16]

Case 5. Long segments

66-year-old man. Ex-smoker; high cholesterol. Mild angina; at Bruce protocol ETT developed mild angina with lateral ST segment depression.

Catheter findings: Moderate overall LV function; long segment of moderate stenosis in mid-LAD; occluded RCA proximally which cross-filled from LCA.

Procedure: JR4 8F guide; 0.014″ high torque intermediate wire backed up by 3.0 mm over-the-wire balloon. Long subintimal course taken by wire, eventually re-entering the true lumen just before the bifurcation.
Stents then deployed as follows:
RCA before bifurcation: (a) Guidant Duet® 3.5 mm × 38 mm; (b) Cordis CrossFlex™ 3.5 mm × 25 mm; (c) Guidant Duet 3.0 mm × 38 mm.
LV branch: (a) Cordis CrossFlex™ 3.0 mm × 15 mm; (b) Cordis CrossFlex™ 3.0 mm × 15 mm Bifurcation of LV branch: (a) Cordis CrossFlex™ 3.0 mm × 15 mm; 1200 ml of contrast. Abciximab (ReoPro®) given at end.

William D Knopf:

The fifth case represents total reconstruction of an occluded right coronary artery. Several key points are illustrated. Most importantly, the guidewire went subintimally and then re-entered the lumen distally. In these circumstances, a distal injection is mandatory to ensure distal wire position and the entire artery must be stented to reconstruct a new lumen. There is clearly diffuse disease in the LV branch as well. This is appropriately stented. Once the stents are placed, a very large vessel is apparent. Optimally sizing the stents again becomes difficult. I favour oversizing the stents with 3.5 mm and 4.0 mm balloons or using IVUS to confirm deployment. Self-expanding or balloon expandable stents may be used. Although the restenosis rate may be high, it may return in a focal manner and be easily retreated. A IIb/IIIa inhibitor is used to help ensure acute and possible long term patency. Given the extent of disease and numbers of stents, I agree with this approach, although there are no definitive data to support its use.

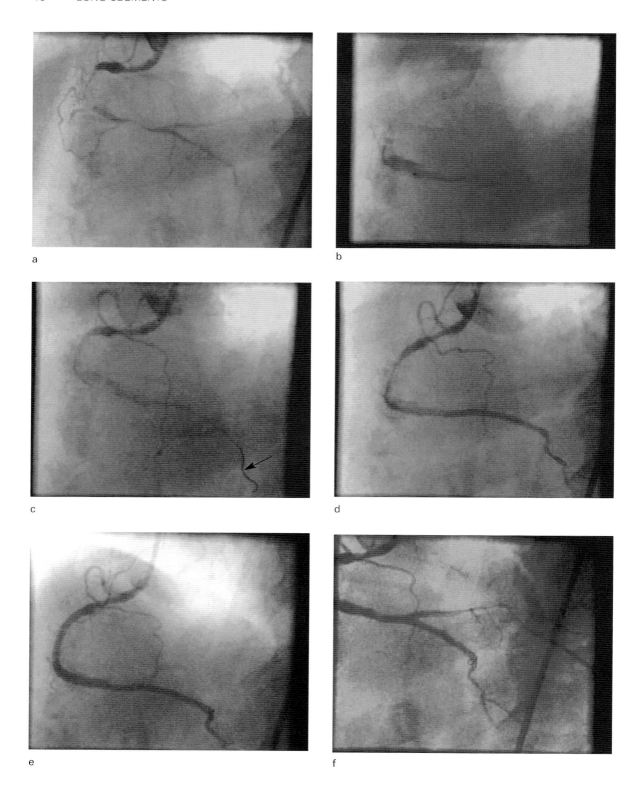

a

b

c

d

e

f

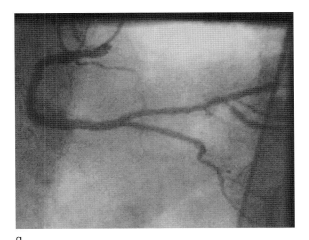

g

Figure 2.7a–g
RCA angiogram. a) Extensive disease from proximal RCA. b) Contrast in false lumen created by guidewire, contrast delivered via over-the-wire balloon. c) Guidewire located to PDA (arrow). d) After dilatation and distal stenting. e) After complete stenting of RCA, note absence of posterior LV branches. f) Posterior LV branches recovered after guidewire passage through side of stent at RCA/PDA junction. g) Final result.

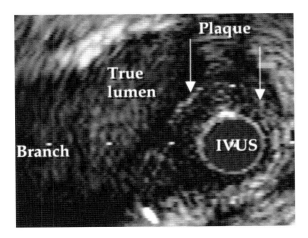

Figure 2.8
IVUS catheter surrounded by plaque (arrows). Side branch off another lumen (see text).

Atsushi Takagi and Peter J Fitzgerald:

Manipulation of a guidewire across a tight or occluded lesion may result in the creation of an extraluminal path. Attempting to dilate a false lumen may result in poor flow or a 'complete jail' of a side branch by an endothelial barrier. Angiography contributes little information to pinpoint the entry and extent of the false lumen. IVUS can often elucidate the exact wire path, and may help to assess the extent of branch jeopardy. Fig. 2.8, below, demonstrates the IVUS catheter surrounded by a cradle of plaque, and a branch which emerged from another lumen. These findings suggest that the guidewire is located in the false lumen. Additionally, simultaneous IVUS observation may be helpful to rewire in this case. Placing the IVUS transducer at the bifurcation, and simultaneously determining the direction of the guidewire aimed into the postero-lateral branch may improve the success in cannulating the true lumen.

Another issue is the timing of abciximab administration. Pharmacological intervention with anti-platelet/anti-coagulation agents prior to the procedure may potentially decrease the incidence of vascular complication and subsequently save the overall cost during the treatment of complex coronary lesions. In order to maximally benefit from abciximab, it should be used 'up-front' rather than after extensive catheter manipulation and the development of poor distal run off.

References

1. Tenaglia A, Zidar J, Jackman J, et al. Treatment of long coronary artery narrowings with long angioplasty balloon catheters. Am J Cardiol 1993;71:1274–1277.
2. Kornowski R, Mehran R, Lansky A, et al. Procedural results and late clinical outcomes following percutaneous interventions using long (≥ 25 mm) stents. J Am Coll Cardiol 1999;33(Suppl A):69A(abstract).
3. Nakagawa Y, Yufu K, Tamura T, et al. Stenting for long lesion with long GFX stent. J Am Coll Cardiol 1999;33(Suppl A):69A(abstract).
4. Kobayashi N, Finci L, Ferraro M, et al. Results of coronary stenting with expanded indications J Am Coll Cardiol 1999;33(Suppl A):68A(abstract).

5. Mehran R, Hong M, Lansky A, et al. Vessel size and lesion length influence late clinical outcomes after native coronary artery stent placement. Circulation 1997;96(Suppl I):1520.

6. Silva J, White C, Gregorio J, et al. Point-counter. Coronary stent implantation in long diffuse or focal sequential lesions: full coverage or spot stenting? Intl J Cardiovasc Intervent 1998;1:113–119.

7. Hong M, Mintz G, Satler L, et al. Full lesion stent coverage reduces subsequent target lesion revascularization: an intravascular ultrasound study. J Am Coll Cardiol 1999;33(Suppl A):61A(abstract).

8. Henneke KH, et al. Impact of target lesion calcification on coronary stent expansion after rotational atherectomy. Am Heart J 1999;137:93.

9. Mintz GS, et al. Determinants and correlates of target lesion calcium in coronary artery disease: a clinical angiographic and intravascular ultrasound study. J Am Coll Cardiol 1997;29:268.

10. Osterle SN, et al. Ultra-sound logic: the value of intracoronary imaging for interventionist. Cathet Cardiovasc Intervent 1999 in press.

11. Kasaoka S, et al. Angiographic and intravascular ultrasound predictors of in-stent restenosis. J Am Coll Cardiol 1998;32:1630.

12. De Gregorio J, et al. A matched comparison between spot stenting and traditional stenting for the treatment of long lesions. J Am Coll Cardiol 1999;33:33A(abstract).

13. Hong MK, et al. In-vivo intravascular ultrasound measured stent lengths do not predict subsequent target lesion revascularization. J Am Coll Cardiol 1999;33:101A(abstract).

14. Moussa I, et al. Does the specific intravascular ultrasound criterion used to optimize stent expansion have an impact on the probability of stent restenosis? Am J Cardiol 1999;83:1012.

15. Kobayashi Y, et al. Relationship between radial expansile force and neointimal proliferation in self-expandable stents: a serial intravascular ultrasound study. Circulation 1998;17:l163(abstract).

16. Pitt B, et al. Aggressive lipid-lowering therapy compared with angioplasty in stable coronary artery disease. N Engl J Med 1999;341:70.

3
Multiple vessels

Percutaneous treatment of multiple vessel coronary disease involves a wide range of technical skills and raises some taxing questions regarding strategy.

- Once it has been decided that a particular case should be treated by angioplasty, should all the vessels be treated at the same sitting or as part of staged procedures?
- If one of the major coronary arteries is occluded and cross-fills from a vessel with significant disease, is it safe to start only by trying to open the occluded vessel?
- Is multivessel stenting an indication for abciximab therapy?
- Should we be inclined to accept incomplete revascularization as a strategy?
- Should we anticipate higher restenosis rates for these cases?
- When a patient presents with an acute history and is found to have multivessel disease is there any indication to treat any lesion apart from the 'culprit' on that occasion?
- Is there, or should there be, an upper limit to the amount of contrast agent and the amount of radiation that should be employed during one sitting in the catheter laboratory?
- What should limit the length of a procedure?

In this chapter we ask **Ulrich Sigwart** and **Carl Brookes** to comment on the management of multivessel disease cases

Case 1. Multiple vessels

56-year-old female. Hypertension; hypercholesterolaemia, ex-smoker. Myocardial infarct April 1996 with mild angina.

Catheter findings: Moderate LV function; non-dominant RCA; LAD and circumflex disease.

Procedure: January 1997
(a) Circumflex: JL4 8F guide; 0.014″ high torque floppy wire. Pre-dilatation with 3.0 mm monorail balloon. Overlapping stents: (i) ACS MULTI-LINK® 3.5 mm × 25 mm; (ii) Cordis Crossflex™ 3.5 mm × 15 mm.
(b) LAD: JL4 8F guide; 0.014″ high torque floppy wire. Pre-dilatation with 3.0 mm monorail balloon. Overlapping stents: (i) ACS MULTI-LINK® 3.5 mm × 15 mm; (ii) ACS MULTI-LINK® 3.0 mm × 25 mm and ACS MULTI-LINK® 3.5 mm × 15 mm in first diagonal branch.

Ulrich Sigwart and Carl Brookes:

This is a case of two vessel disease with a very tight circumflex lesion and long tubular LAD stenosis. In the elective setting both vessels could be done in one session as neither lesion is particularly complex. This is not a case for a staged procedure as everything can be done with one guiding catheter and it would not necessarily be a long procedure. In general, the radiation dose and the contrast load are the two main factors that govern whether or not we would perform a staged procedure.

As with most cases of multiple vessel intervention we would start with the tightest lesion—in this case the circumflex. We would probably not have placed the distal stent to the bifurcation of the AV branch of the circumflex as the disease in the distal portion does not seem to be very severe. Instead, we would have placed only one long stent in the circumflex and probably would have chosen the ACS MULTI-LINK® as well. We would have tackled the LAD in much the same way but doubt whether we would have treated the diagonal. Using this strategy three stents and not five would have been used.

In the acute/unstable setting we would have done the circumflex alone and come back to do the LAD in another session. Abciximab is not automatically necessary in such a case but we would use it if we anticipated thrombotic problems.

We have some doubts about long term results with the Cordis CrossFlex™ stent as the coil structure may increase the risk of plaque protrusion, resulting in higher rates of restenosis.

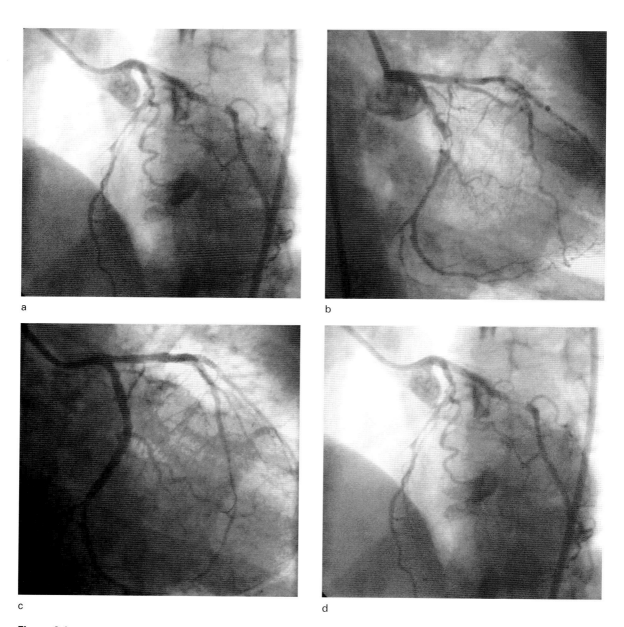

a

b

c

d

Figure 3.1
LCA angiogram. a,b) Lesions seen in main Cx and mid-LAD. c,d) Result after stenting.

Case 2. Multiple vessels

66-year-old woman. IDDM; hypercholesterol-aemia. CABG surgery 1996 (left internal mammary artery [LIMA] to LAD, VG to OM). Recurrent angina 1997, admission with unstable angina May 1997.

Catheter findings: Moderate LV; RCA unobstructed; severe stenosis over long segment of LAD; OM1 occluded; OM2 stenosed; VG to OM patent; LIMA patent.

Procedure: JL4 (8F) guide.
LAD: 0.014″ high torque floppy wire; extensive pre-dilatation with 3.0 mm monorail balloon. Then stents overlapping length of vessel, from distal to proximal as follows:
(a) AVE Microstent 3.0 mm × 12 mm; (b) Cordis CrossFlex™ 3.0 mm × 15 mm; (c) Cordis CrossFlex™ 3.0 mm × 15 mm; (d) AVE GFX 3.5 mm × 18 mm; (e) AVE Microstent 3.5 mm × 30 mm.
Circumflex: 0.014″ high torque floppy wire. 3.0 mm monorail pre-dilatation, followed by NIR™ 3 mm × 32 mm more distally overlapped by Cordis CrossFlex™ 3.5 mm × 15 mm in the OM.

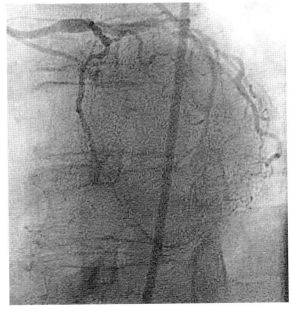

a

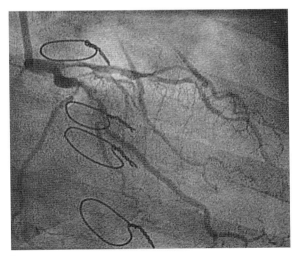

b

Figure 3.2a–e
LCA angiogram. a,b) Extensive disease in LAD from proximal through to distal vessel.

continued

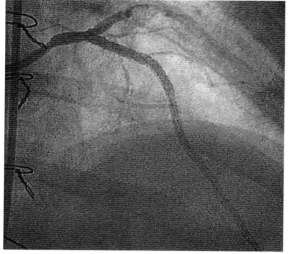

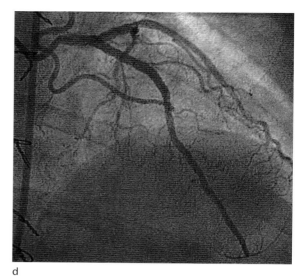

c

d

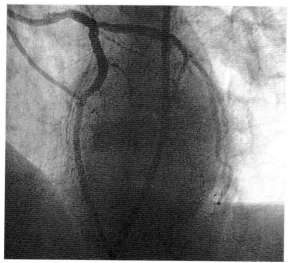

e

Figure 3.2 *continued*
c) Result of LAD stenting. d) After pre-dilatation of Cx. e) Result of extensive stent implantation.

Ulrich Sigwart and Carl Brookes:

This is a case of extensive left coronary artery disease after previous bypass surgery. One graft to the first obtuse marginal branch is patent as is the LIMA to the LAD.

The most severe lesion is probably the lesion of the second OM branch and we would treat this first. This lesion could be covered by one long stent (about 25 mm to 35 mm long). We would have left the ostium of the AV circumflex alone as well.

The LAD may or may not benefit from angioplasty. As the LIMA insertion appears to be fine and the distal vessel does not seem to be significantly diseased we would probably leave it alone. This becomes important because of the involvement of the proximal LAD almost to the point of the LIMA anastamosis. If everything were treated as described in this case the LIMA would be stent-jailed. A conservative management plan for this vessel would, in our opinion, be appropriate, particularly as the only data showing improved survival relate to the patency of IMA grafts.

The operators have deployed seven stents in this patient and according to our approach we would have used only one.

The other issue that arises from this case is whether one can place stents from different manufacturers side by side or even overlapping and this is a question that nobody has resolved yet. If the same material is used (in this case 316L stainless steel) local elements should, in theory, not play a role.

Case 3. Multiple vessels

60-year-old man. Ex-smoker; hypercholesterol-aemia; hypertension. PTCA with J+J stent to proximal LAD two years previously. Recurrent angina.

Catheter findings: RCA blocked at origin of PDA; circumflex occluded; significant disease in mid-LAD beyond previous stent.

Procedure:
LAD: JL4 (8F) guide; 0.014″ high torque floppy wire. 3.0 mm monorail balloon, then ACS MULTI-LINK® 3.5 mm × 25 mm to 12 atm, overlapping distal end of previous stent.
Circumflex: Attempted disobliteration using 0.014″ high torque floppy wire backed by 1.5 mm over-the-wire balloon—unsuccessful.

Ulrich Sigwart and Carl Brookes:

Again a case of advanced left coronary artery disease involving the circumflex and the LAD. The right coronary artery appears to be blocked as well, although the degree of cross-filling is not well seen. The right coronary artery occlusion, of course, poses a certain threat to any procedure, particularly as the collaterals to the right coronary artery appear to leave from the circumflex (AV branch) as well as from the LAD. The LAD has one tight stenosis which should not create too many problems, the circumflex artery, however, is technically very difficult.

We would tend to send this patient for surgery if there were no concomitant medical problems. In treating the LAD alone, not only would this represent incomplete revascularization but also the placement of a stent in this territory may interfere with the later insertion of an IMA graft. As the patient is very likely to come to need CABG we would probably refrain from doing anything and submit him to surgical revascularization.

Incomplete revascularization is not necessarily a contraindication to percutaneous intervention, especially in the acute setting, but on balance, this patient is likely to get much better symptomatic relief from CABG.

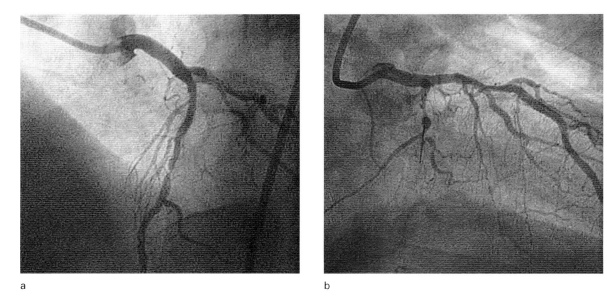

a   b

Figure 3.3
LCA angiogram. a) Extensive LAD disease with tight mid-LAD lesion. b) After stenting of LAD. The disobliteration of circumflex has been attempted without result.

Case 4. Multiple vessels

76-year-old woman. Ex-smoker. Poorly differentiated squamous cell carcinoma of the right lung requiring urgent surgery. Angina on exertion with abnormal ETT.

Catheter findings: Moderate LV with inferior hypokinesis; significant stenosis in RCA (dominant); further disease in LAD.

First procedure: JL4 8F guide; 0.014″ high torque floppy wire; pre-dilatation with 3.0 mm monorail balloon. Cordis CrossFlex™ 3.0 mm × 15 mm deployed just after diagonal origin.
Three days later presented with anterior ST elevation and pain. Catheter showed stent occlusion and nipping of diagonal origin. Therefore:

Second Procedure:
LAD/D1: JL4 8F guide; 0.014″ high torque floppy wire; pre-dilatation within stent using 3.0 mm monorail balloon. Then 'Y' stent fashioned using further Cordis CrossFlex™ 3.5 mm × 15 mm stent across origin of diagonal and Cordis CrossFlex™ 3.0 mm × 15 mm into diagonal from LAD.
RCA: JR4 (8F); 0.014″ high torque floppy wire. Pre-dilatation with 3.0 mm monorail balloon, then 3.5 mm × 25 mm Cordis CrossFlex™ stent.

Ulrich Sigwart and Carl Brookes:

This is a case of significant two-vessel coronary disease with intervention based on the avoidance of general anaesthetic in a patient urgently in need of surgery for cancer.

As mentioned above, it is our usual practice to tackle the more difficult lesion first and we would therefore attempt the right coronary lesion before the LAD at the first sitting. It is difficult to comment on the results of the LAD angioplasty, as we do not see the films prior to stent insertion. It would also have been helpful to know whether the patient was given aggressive antiplatelet therapy after the first stenting.

We would probably have used a long stent in the LAD, jailing the diagonal vessel, as there is clearly disease proximal to the origin of the first diagonal artery. If we were concerned about losing the diagonal vessel we may have placed a second wire down this vessel before stenting the LAD to act as a geographical marker for access. There are clearly problems of fashioning a Y stent, as the chances of restenosis in this vessel will be high. The result in the RCA looks good.

In general our rules for the use of abciximab is in cases of clinical instability or where there is evidence of thrombus formation or dissection within the coronary arteries. At present we do not see there being a role for abciximab purely on the basis of the number of stents inserted.

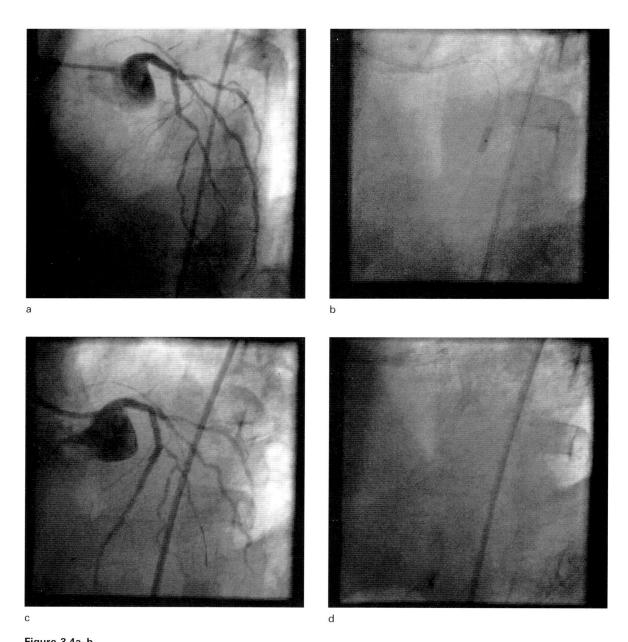

Figure 3.4a–h
LCA angiogram. a) Extensive disease in tortuous LAO. b) Guidewire down LAD. c) After LAD balloon and stenting. Diagonal ostial stenosis to a possibly large vessel. d) True Y stent in LAD/diagonal junction.

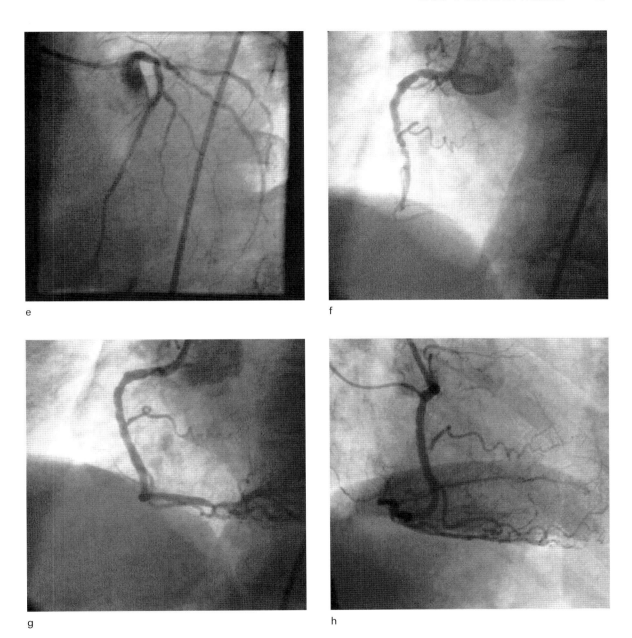

Figure 3.4 *continued*
e) Result in LAD. Good result in both LAD and diagonal origin. f) Occluded distal RCA. g,h) Result after disobliteration and stent implantation.

4
Total chronic occlusions

Total chronic occlusions present unique challenges. The symptomatic benefits of success are often very great but even in the most competent hands they have a considerably lower procedural success rate than perhaps any other lesion type in intervention. Even angiographic features that predict success to one cardiologist may not to another! Procedure strategy, especially choice of guide catheter, guidewire and balloon are considered to be critical factors. There has been a considerable body of data published recently to suggest unequivocal benefit for the stenting of a successfully angioplastied chronically occluded segment.

Common questions

- Should the chosen guide catheter be more aggressive in terms of ostial engagement and support than for other lesions?
- Is the over-the-wire approach superior because of guidewire support, ability to exchange guidewires without loss of position, and the capacity to inject to test for luminal position?
- Should the initial guidewire be stiffer than normal or hydrophilic?
- Is it valuable to assess cross-filling from the other coronary simultaneously?
- Is there a place for other technologies such as laser?
- When is the right time to admit defeat?

Ian M Penn was asked to comment on these cases of chronic total occlusion.

Case 1. Total chronic occlusions

40-year-old man. Smoker; family history. Inferior MI June 1996. Exertional angina May 1997.

Catheter findings: Good overall LV with mild inferior hypokinesis; left coronary artery unobstructed; RCA as shown.

Procedure: JR4 (8F) guide with sideholes; 0.014" high torque floppy wire. 2.5 mm monorail for pre-dilatation then Wallstent® 4.5 mm × 47 mm overlapped by Wallstent® 5.0 mm × 31 mm proximally. Post-deployment dilatation with 4.5 mm Chubby™ balloon.

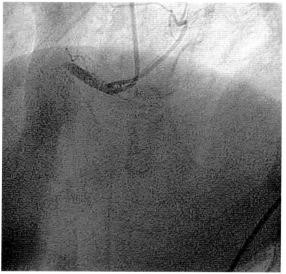

a

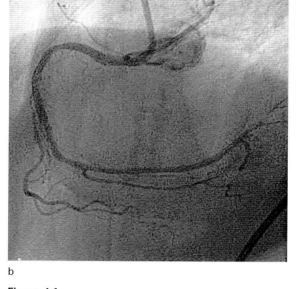

b

Figure 4.1
RCA angiogram. a) Occluded proximal RCA. b) After disobliteration. c) Result.

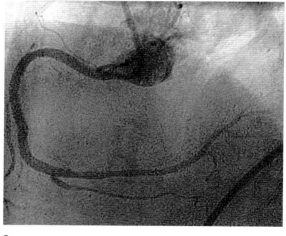

c

Ian M Penn:

Although this occlusion is over a year old, the appearance on the angiogram, that of haziness with no major collaterals or side branches beyond the conus branch, is of a recent occlusion. This is consistent with a recanalized right coronary artery post-infarction and exertional angina due to re-occlusion of this vessel.

Although the JR4 is a reasonable first choice, in the presence of outgoing or horizontal take-off an Amplatz AL1 or a 'hockey stick' can provide more coaxial support against the posterior wall of the aorta. The fact that this was crossed with a high torque floppy wire again is suggestive of recent re-occlusion of a recanalized RCA.

The choice in length of stent is still controversial. Restenosis is dependent on both lesion length and stent length. Spot stenting of a focal disease has been associated with good long-term angiographic results. It is usual, however, in total occlusion to have a longer area of disease than is angiographically apparent and therefore a longer stent is probably wise. Here a long Wallstent® is applied with good angiographic paving. Balloon dilatation only in the presence of a chronic total occlusion has been associated with a high angiographic restenosis rate. This clinical history would probably also confirm the work by Zilstra showing the higher incidence of late re-intervention in patients treated with thrombolytics vs. PTCA in acute myocardial infarction.

Case 2. Total chronic occlusions

38-year-old man. Hypercholesterolaemia; ex-smoker; family history. Severely limiting angina with abnormal ETT.

Catheter findings: Good LV; Proximally occluded dominant RCA; moderate lesion in OM of circumflex.

Procedure: Amplatz Left 2 (8F) guide; standard 0.014" high torque wire, initially backed up by 1.5 mm over-the-wire balloon. Extensive subintimal course of wire accepted with re-entry into

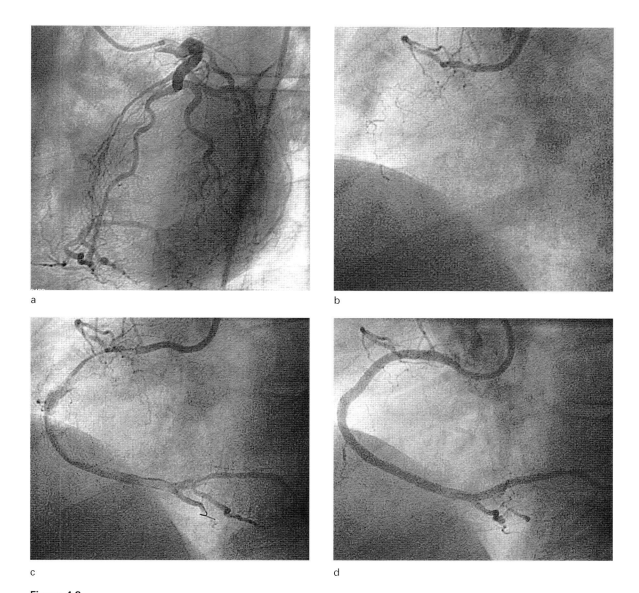

a

b

c

d

Figure 4.2
LCA angiogram. a) Collateral to RCA. b) Occluded proximal RCA. c) Dissected RCA after wire passage and balloon inflation. d) Result.

true lumen (confirmed by contrast injection down central lumen of over-the-wire balloon at junction with PDA). Further dilatation of path taken by wire using 3.0 mm monorail balloon. Overlapping stents from distal to proximal as follows:

(a) AVE GFX 3.0 mm × 18 mm; (b) Cordis CrossFlex™ 3.0 mm × 12 mm; (c) ACS MULTI-LINK® 3.5 mm × 35 mm; (d) ACS MULTI-LINK® 4.0 mm × 25 mm; (e) ACS MULTI-LINK® 4.0 mm × 25 mm; (f) 4.0 mm × 25 mm. Abciximab (ReoPro®) bolus plus infusion.

Ian M Penn:

This young patient has a proximal, possibly ostial, occlusion of a dominant right coronary artery. The choice of a strong guide, e.g. Amplatz, and a standard wire shortens the procedure time, with few adverse events in crossing,

most of the complications arising with distal dissection once through the occlusion. The use of an over-the-wire balloon to fortify this would strengthen the initial crossing parameters. This is usually a very safe strategy as the balloon can obtain co-axial movement of the wire into the true lumen. In this case, however, there is extensive subintimal dissection with re-entry proximal to the PDA. Thus, we are presented with a dissected conduit to the origin of the PDA and this needs basically to be treated as an internal graft. This can be accomplished by Wallstent®, or multiple stents, as has been performed in this case with an adequate angiographic result. As long as the outflow is reasonable, especially at the posterior descending branch, the likelihood of early re-occlusion is low. By contrast, the likelihood of restenosis is high, given the degree of dissection. In our experience many patients have been treated adequately in the long term with this approach of re-entry into a true lumen with the deployment of long stents.

Case 3. Total chronic occlusions

55-year-old man. Smoker; family history. Limiting exertional angina.

Catheter findings: March 1997 good LV; occlusion proximal Circumflex; irregularities in LAD and RCA only.

Procedure: Amplatz Left 2 (8F) guide; 0.014″ high torque standard wire to cross lesion backed up by 3.0 mm over-the-wire balloon. Site of occlusion stented with 3.0 mm × 18 mm AVE GFX.

Ian M Penn:

This is a good example of a short occlusion in

a difficult anatomy treated well with stenting. The proximal circumflex occlusion is well addressed with an Amplatz guide. The guiding catheter is critical in this setting as the guidewire loses its strength in crossing with the bend in the circumflex. This is all the more common in occlusions in marginal circumflex branches where several bends are required to be negotiated prior to the occlusion. In this procedure again a high torque standard was used backed-up by an over-the-wire balloon with good recanalization followed by definitive stenting with an AVE GFX stent. This is also a useful choice of stent with open architecture allowing access to a significant marginal side branch should there be encroachment on this branch during the stent placement.

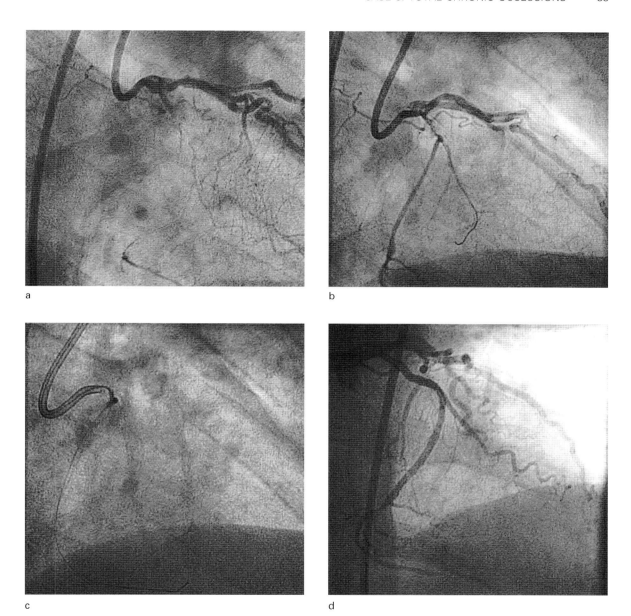

Figure 4.3
LCA angiogram. a) Total proximal occlusion of Cx. b) After balloon dilatation. c) Wire seen in distal branches.
d) Result.

Case 4. Total chronic occlusions

71-year-old male. Ex-smoker; NIDDM. Stable but limiting angina.

Catheter findings: Good LV; proximal LAD occlusion with cross-filling from RCA; no other obstructive disease.

Procedure: JL4 short tip (8F); 0.014″ high torque floppy wire with 1.5 mm over-the-wire balloon for back-up and initial dilatation. Monorail 3.0 mm balloon followed by 3.0 mm × 18 mm AVE GFX stent.

Ian M Penn:

Here is a characteristic example of a recent occlusion to a proximal left anterior descending artery, usually a straight segment, with a hazy distal angiographic appearance. Crossing of this could be anticipated with a softer wire but again this is fortified by the use of an over-the-wire balloon for back-up and pre-dilatation. The final angiographic result is acceptable.

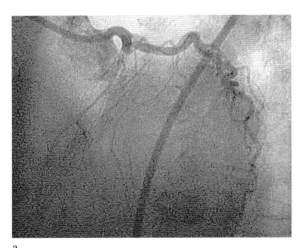

a

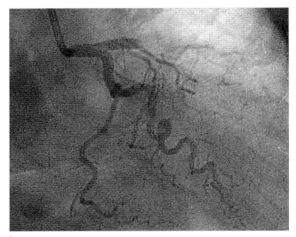

b

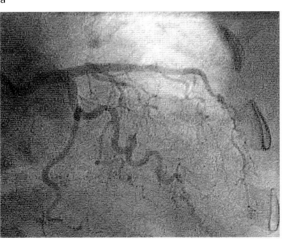

c

Figure 4.4
LCA angiogram. a,b) Total occlusion of proximal LAD. c) Result.

Case 5. Total chronic occlusions

51-year-old man. Hypercholesterolaemia; family history. CABG surgery 1995: LIMA to LAD; vein grafts to RCA, OM, intermediate, diagonal. Presented with unstable angina.

Catheter findings: LV moderate; occlusion of proximal LAD; severe stenoses in circumflex and intermediate vessels; native RCA occluded after RV branch and cross-filling from LCA; RCA graft occluded; LIMA, VGs to OM and intermediate patent.

Procedure: JR4 (8F) guide; 0.014" high torque intermediate wire backed up by 1.5 mm over-the-wire balloon. Subintimal dissection with no re-entry and ECG changes and pain. Procedure abandoned, creatinine kinase (CK) peak of 675 IU.

Ian M Penn:

This is a more difficult procedure involving an old occlusion of the right coronary artery with a web of collaterals coming off the right coronary artery and also collaterals from the left system indicating both chronicity of the occlusion and a lowering of the success rate.

The use of a 0.014" intermediate wire backed-up by a 1.5 mm over-the-wire system is a reasonable initial approach. This provides tip control rather than blind poking. In this case, it was unsuccessful with inability to re-enter the true lumen. This may well relate to vessel tortuosity beyond the occlusion point or the entry into a false channel at the ostium. The patient developed chest pain and ECG changes, consistent with myocardial or alternatively pericardial involvement. In post CABG patients, it is not uncommon to have a thickened pericardial region and it can increase the risk of dissection in the AV groove portion of the right coronary artery.

This is a good example of where guide support would be required. When one sees the horizontal take-off in the LAO projection with a posterior direction in the RAO, it is unusual for a JR4 to fit well and provide good back-up. In this setting, some form of extra support guide, such as AL1 or 'hockey stick' would be a good start.

This case also brings up for discussion how to find your way in a blind pouch. The use of careful prodding with a low profile but torqueable wire, and passage of a low-profile balloon without pre-dilatation is a reasonable approach. The presence of extra systoles, ST segment elevation, chest pain or hypotension due to extra vascular passage of the wire should prompt termination of this passage. It is unusual to require a covered stent for this form of perforation as these usually self-heal.

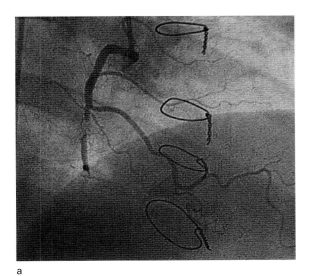

a

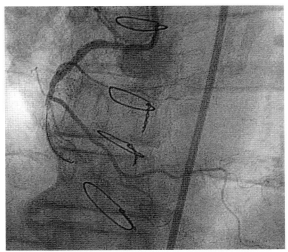

b

Figure 4.5
RCA angiogram. a) Mid-RCA lesion with bridge collaterals to give antegrade flow. Total occlusion distally. b) Guidewire through stented lesion but not through distal occlusion.

Case 6. Total chronic occlusions

63-year-old man. Hypercholesterolaemia; family history. Limiting exertional angina. Inferolateral ST segment depression at 4 minutes Bruce ETT.

Catheter findings: Good LV; LCA unobstructed; RCA occluded as shown.

Procedure: JR4 (8F) guide; 0.014″ high torque floppy wire backed up by 3.0 mm over-the-wire balloon. Then two ACS MULTI-LINK® 3.5 mm × 12 mm stents with a small gap between them.

Ian M Penn:

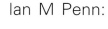

This is an example of a recent occlusion recanalized well by a soft wire with extra back-up with an over-the-wire balloon.

This case exemplifies the question of the use of short versus long stents on the straightened portion of the right coronary artery. It is my practice to try and use a longer stent in this setting to provide good streamlined coverage and take up any distal tears that are not evident angiographically. In this case, there is a gap between the two, evident angiographically. This could be a site of early or late occlusion or restenosis.

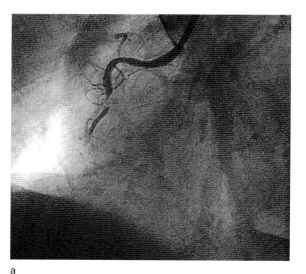

a

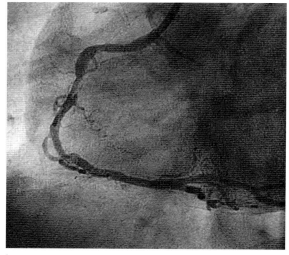

b

Figure 4.6
RCA angiogram. a) Mid-RCA stenosis with mid-vessel total occlusion. b) Vessel opened, local dissection of stenotic site. c) Final result.

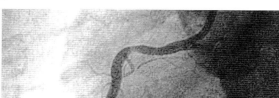

c

Case 7. Total chronic occlusions

69-year-old. Ex-smoker; hypercholesterolaemia. Rapid onset exertional angina.

Catheter findings: Good LV; occluded LAD; RCA and circumflex unobstructed.

Procedure: Amplatz Left 2; 0.014" wire backed up by 1.5 mm over-the-wire balloon. Wire would only enter a diagonal artery. Procedure abandoned.

Ian M Penn:

This is an example of a recent occlusion to the left anterior descending with the stump having abrupt hazy cut-off, distal to the first septal perforator and diagonal.

This area of the left anterior descending is often tortuous and although there is a high chance of success in the proximal LAD occlusion (proximal to the first diagonal) the incidence of success drops in this setting. This relates to vessel tortuosity, the presence of side branches, and the possibility of disease in the segments.

In this case, the wire is able to enter a diagonal and the procedure was abandoned. I am unsure as to why the diagonal alone was not opened. Occasionally this can provide access into the LAD in the setting of an occlusion that goes from the left anterior descending to the diagonal, improving visibility of and access to the ongoing left anterior descending. If the diagonal is a small branch, however, this is unlikely to result in any significant improvement.

The mechanism of re-entering the true lumen after entering a false lumen is based on a lot of experience. Things often feel right or wrong based upon free movement of the distal wire tip. I tend to use a stiffer wire with a short tip that allows me to see the continued free movement of the wire and direct it into branches at will. I favour a BMW wire or a 0.014" intermediate or standard for crossing the original occlusion. If this does not cross, I will go to a hydrophilic wire (Cross-IT™) which has both good tip control as well as ability to penetrate somewhat dense occlusions. Failure to cross an occlusion would prompt me to use a Shinobi wire, which I use in

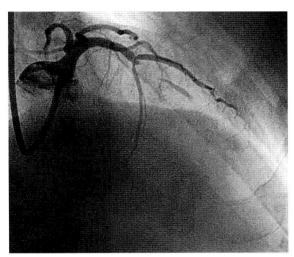

a

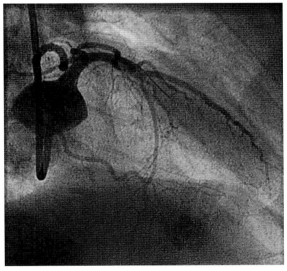

b

Figure 4.7
LCA angiogram. a) Mid-stenosis and then total occlusion. b) Wire through stenosis but not into distal vessel.

increasing strengths. This wire, again, has a hydrophilic coating, has excellent tip control, but is well able to dissect and create new lumens unless care is used in movement.

Case 8. Total chronic occlusions

68-year-old man. Ex-smoker; family history; hyper-cholesterolaemia. Limiting exertional angina.

Catheter findings: LV good; unobstructed RCA cross-filling LAD; LAD occluded after first diagonal; tight proximal diagonal stenosis.

Procedure: Left Voda 3.5 (8F) guide; 0.014" high torque floppy wire; 2.5 mm monorail balloon to proximal diagonal lesion—not stented, considered too small. LAD could not be disobliterated.

Ian M Penn:

Here is a good example of the complexity of the left anterior descending beyond the first diagonal. Again, you can see the angulation of the left anterior descending and in this lesion the chronicity of the total occlusion due to the stub ending at the site of the first septal perforator. The chance of crossing this is extremely low in the absence of any stub to gain purchase on the left anterior descending.

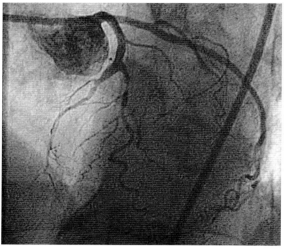

a

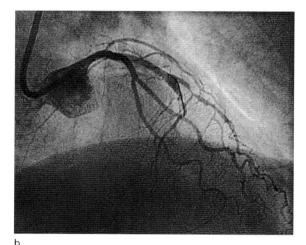

b

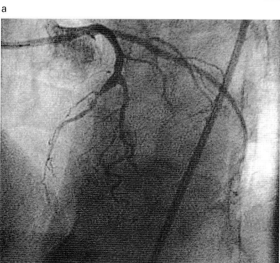

c

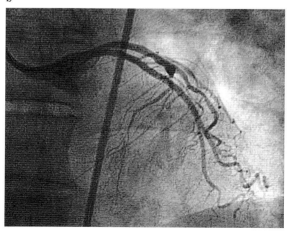

d

Figure 4.8
LCA angiogram. a,b) Mid-LAD to extensive distal vessel disease, and diagonal disease. c,d) Diagonal dilated, LAD not dealt with.

Case 9. Total chronic occlusions

66-year-old man. Hypertension; family history. Presented with limiting exertional angina. Diagnostic cardiac catheter 10 weeks before this admission showed good LV and severe, discrete stenosis of LAD just after origin of first diagonal.

Catheter now: LAD occluded and cross-filling from RCA.

Procedure: Right femoral artery 8F sheath. JL4 (8F) guide; 0.014″ high torque floppy wire. Attempt to disobliterate LAD hampered by wire passing into branches. Eventually wire advanced, but not running forward and therefore unclear whether it was in LAD or not. Therefore, 6F sheath introduced into left femoral artery. JR4 catheter used for RCA injection and retrograde filling of LAD seen, confirming appropriate direction of wire. Inflation at occlusion point with 2.5 mm over-the-wire balloon in LAD. Next shot shows 'saddle embolus' in bifurcation of large diagonal (Fig. 4.9e). Cordis CrossFlex™ 3.0 mm × 15 mm stent deployed in LAD to 12 atm. Good result in LAD; some thrombus still visible in diagonal at end. Abciximab (ReoPro®) bolus and infusion.

Ian M Penn:

Here is a good case of the use of multiple injections, and contralateral injections to confirm position in an LAD occlusion. The diagonal is patent and some sense of the distal LAD is given in the second injection (Figure 4.9d). During the procedure, cross-talk may well have occurred, resulting in inability of the wire to move forward. The angiographic appearance in Fig. 4.9e is consistent with a saddle embolus but it is also consistent with intimal disruption due to wire manipulation at the occlusion site. Fortunately this was treated with a CrossFlex™ stent with some distal narrowing and haziness. The likelihood of improved benefit by further stenting is low and therefore ReoPro® has been used in this setting. The basis for this use is an extension of the data from the EPILOG and EPISTENT investigations in which ReoPro® was presumed to have an improved clinical outcome in the setting of distal dissection.

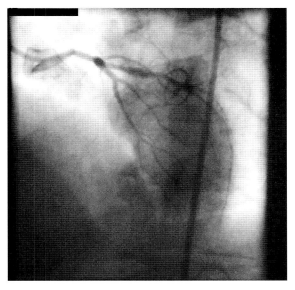

a

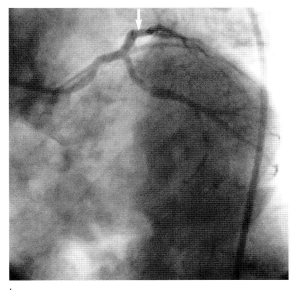

b

Figure 4.9a–f
LCA angiogram. a-c) Occluded LAD, stump seen at arrow, line of LAD not clear from these views.

continued

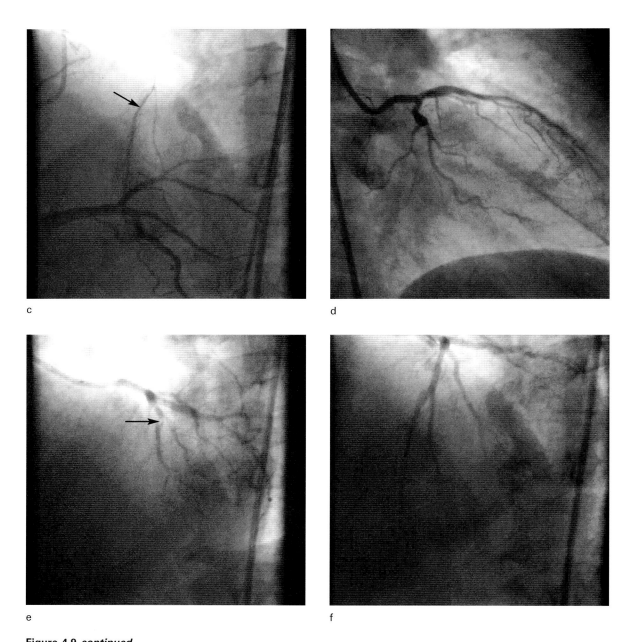

Figure 4.9 *continued*
d) RCA injection with delayed filling of distal LAD. Guidewire seen to be in LAD, at arrow. e) LAD dilated but clot seen at arrow. f) Result after balloon and stenting.

Case 10. Total chronic occlusions

35-year-old man. Smoker; high cholesterol; family history. Limiting angina following inferior MI 18 months before.

Catheter findings: Moderate LV function with inferior hypokinesis; moderate lesion in mid LAD; occlusion of PDA branch of RCA.

Procedure: JR4 8F guide; 0.014″ high torque floppy wire backed up with 2.5 mm over-the-wire balloon for disobliteration and pre-dilatation. Guidant Duet 3.5 mm × 12 mm.

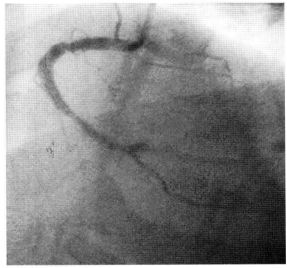

a

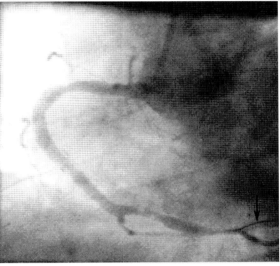

b

Figure 4.10
RCA angiogram. a) Distal occlusion in posterior LV branch. b) After disobliteration, wire seen in posterior LV branch (arrow). c) Result.

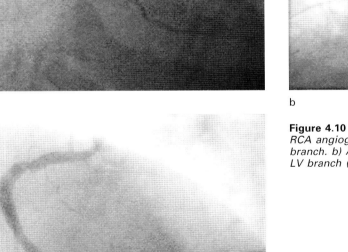

c

Case 11. Total chronic occlusions

68-year-old man. High cholesterol. Stable, limiting angina.

Catheter findings: Unobstructed LCA; occlusion of RCA; good LV.

Procedure: JR4 8F guide; 0.014″ high torque floppy wire backed up with 1.5 mm over-the-wire balloon. Then pre-dilatation with 3.0 mm monorail balloon followed by AVE GFX 3.0 mm × 18 mm.

Ian M Penn:

These are good examples of scaffolding in short occlusion.

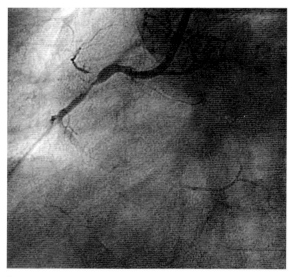

a

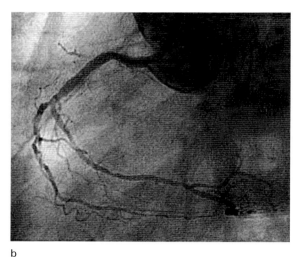

b

Figure 4.11
RCA angiogram. a) Proximal RCA stenosis and slow, poor flow distally through occlusion. b) Result.

5
Bifurcation disease

The treatment of bifurcation lesions is the subject of considerable investigation and controversy. It has been established that balloon angioplasty alone is often associated with a poor angiographic outcome and risk of occlusion or restenosis in one of the three limbs of the bifurcation. A myriad of different stenting strategies have therefore emerged that aim to improve immediate and long term outcomes. These stent configurations are described as 'T', 'Y', 'true Y', 'culottes' and 'monoclonal antibody'. It is clear, however, that the definitive technique has not yet been determined and the suspicion that the more complex stent formations may be associated with high restenosis rates remains to be clarified. Manufacturers meanwhile continue to search for a user-friendly and effective 'ready-to-use' tailor-made bifurcation stent. That there is not a single interventional solution to all such cases is clear cut.

Common decisions

- Should both limbs be wired early?
- Does a stent down one arm trap the other wire in a dangerous fashion?
- Which stents should not be used if the intention is to balloon through the side of the stent?
- Should kissing balloons be routine at the end of the procedure?
- Should IVUS be routine?

Marie-Claude Morice and **Antonio Colombo** were asked to comment on a selection of bifurcation cases.

Marie-Claude Morice makes these general comments before considering the cases

Management of bifurcation lesions at the Institut Cardiovasculaire Paris Sud (ICPS) involves prior analysis of the type of bifurcation to be treated according to the classification into four lesion types (Fig. 5.1), as defined by our team. Treatment is selected following lesion analysis.

We routinely use a 6F large lumen guiding catheter (Zuma, Medtronic or Viking, Guidant). Kissing balloon dilatation can be performed through such guiding catheters even with 2 × 3.5 mm balloons (with Viva balloons only).

Lesion classification: morphology

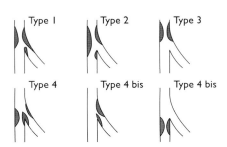

Treatment classification

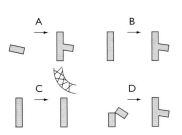

Figure 5.1
Bifurcation classification and treatment classification.

Case 1. Bifurcation disease

59-year-old man. High cholesterol; positive family history. Limiting exertional angina.

Catheter findings: Good LV; single vessel disease of LAD.

Procedure: JL4 (8F); 0.014″ high torque floppy wire. 3.0 mm monorail balloon followed by Medtronic Wiktor® 3.5 mm × 16 mm to 10 atm across origin of D1 (the first diagonal) in LAD, no treatment to the diagonal.

Marie-Claude Morice:

According to the lesion classification used at the ICPS, this is a 4b type lesion for which treatment D would have been selected. In this case, I would not have used a protective guidewire in the diagonal either, since the vessel was disease-free and easily accessible even if the balloon subsequently caused diagonal ostial deterioration. I would have used a short stent (short tubular type such as Guidant Duet or Scimed-Boston NIR™) in the LAD lesion implanted just distal to the diagonal. If deterioration of the diagonal ostium had occurred, I would have performed a kissing balloon dilatation with a 3.5 mm balloon in the LAD and a 3.0 mm balloon without stent in the diagonal using two Viva balloons which can be inserted together in a 6F guiding catheter.

Editors: It is interesting that Dr Morice would consider the NIR™ even though she acknowledges that she may need to go through the side of it if the diagonal is compromised. Our belief, which is certainly supported by some data, is that the cells of the NIR™ are not well suited to the trauma of a balloon inflation within them. Therefore, we tend to avoid the NIR™ if there is the possibility of requiring side branch access.

Antonio Colombo:

The strategy to stent the major branch with the Wiktor® stent is quite appropriate because this type of stent has been used with success in the treatment of bifurcational disease.[1,2] The first diagonal may require simple balloon dilatation. Our strategy

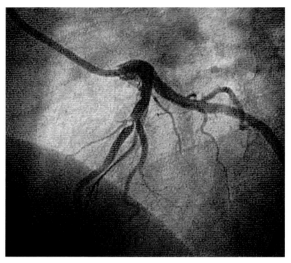

a

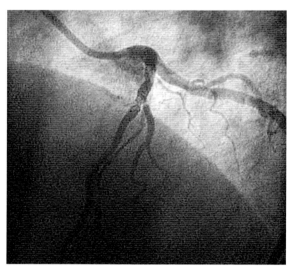

b

Figure 5.2
LCA angiogram. a) Lesion at LAD/diagonal junction. b) Result.

is to perform a pre-dilatation of the diagonal before deploying the stent into the LAD if the origin of the diagonal is compromised. The wire will then be removed from the diagonal and the stent in the LAD will be deployed. The diagonal will be dilated again if significant compromise is present. A stent will be deployed in the diagonal only to treat abrupt closure or threatened closure.

Case 2. Bifurcation disease

56-year-old man. Hypertensive; smoker; family history. Unstable angina with anterior T-wave inversion.

Catheter findings: LV: poor overall function with extensive anteroapical hypokinesis; occluded circumflex; RCA dominant and unobstructed; LAD stenosis involving two large diagonals.

Procedure: JL3.5 (8F); 0.014″ high torque floppy wire to LAD, D1 (the first diagonal) and D2 (the second diagonal). 3.0 mm monorail balloon to LAD followed by 3.5 mm × 15 mm ACS MULTI-LINK® stent in LAD across origin of diagonals. Well-preserved flow in all vessels.

Marie-Claude Morice:

This is a type 2 bifurcation lesion, particularly complex because of the two diagonal branches originating from the lesion, though fortunately disease-free. I would have selected exactly the same treatment, i.e. protecting the two diagonals and performing stenting of the LAD covering the two branches. We would probably have used a beStent™ tubular stent which provides optimal access to the side branches (in our experience non-tubular stents are associated with higher restenosis). Although beStent™ is probably the best choice, MULTI-LINK DUET™ could also be used though providing less optimal access to branches.

Antonio Colombo:

The strategy proposed is quite appropriate. Alternative stents could be the GFX2, the CrossFlex™ LC or the Wiktor® stent. Another approach could be to perform prior debulking with directional atherectomy in the LAD and then proceed as outlined. Preliminary data from our database point out that bifurcational lesions treated with debulking (DCA) followed by stenting are associated with a lower angiographic and clinical recurrence rate.[3]

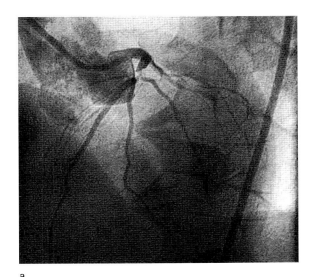

a

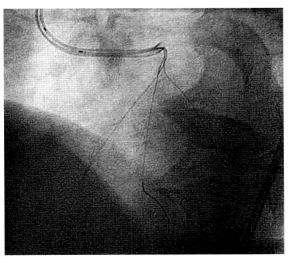

b

Figure 5.3a–e
LCA angiogram. a) Trifurcation lesion. b) 3 guidewires in LAD, diagonals 1 and 2.

continued

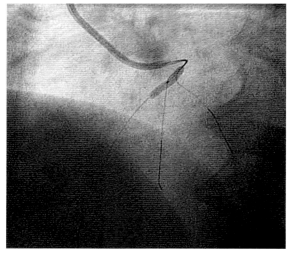

c

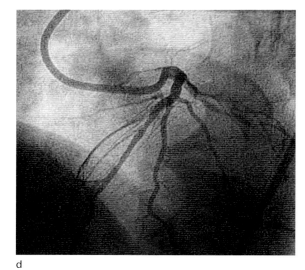

d

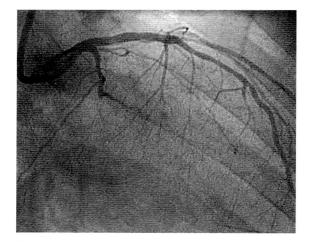

e

Figure 5.3 *continued*
c) Balloon dilatation in lesion with side branch
protection. d,e) Result.

Case 3. Bifurcation disease

43-year-old man. Smoker; high cholesterol; family history. Acute inferior MI treated with streptokinase, with post infarct angina.

Catheter findings: Good LV; tight lesion in dominant RCA; significant LAD stenosis involving origin of large diagonal.

Procedure:
- RCA: JR4 (8F); 0.014″ high torque floppy wire; 3.0 mm monorail balloon; Cordis CrossFlex™ 3.0 mm × 15 mm stent.
- LAD/D1: JL4 (8F). A 'Y' stent was fashioned in steps as follows (Fig. 5.4a–t):
  a. Diagnostic in LAO cranial projection
  b. 0.014″ high torque floppy wires to both LAD and first diagonal (D1)
  c. 3.0 mm monorail balloon inflation in LAD lesion
  d. Result of c
  e. 3.0 mm monorail balloon inflation in D1 lesion
  f. Result of e
  g. 3.0 mm × 15 mm Cordis CrossFlex™ stent in LAD across D1 origin
  h. Result in LAO cranial view
  i. Result in RAO view
  j. Result in LAO caudal view
  k. Pull back D1 wire into proximal LAD and then
  l. Pass it back into D1 through the side of the LAD stent
  m. 2.5 mm monorail balloon inflated through side of LAD stent to 12 atm
  n. Result of m
  o. Position Cordis CrossFlex™ 3.0 mm × 15 mm stent into D1 from LAD via the side of the LAD stent *and pull back LAD wire before inflation*
  p. Result
  q. Result
  r. Pass LAD wire back down LAD through side of D1 stent, and then inflate 2.5 mm monorail balloon through side to 12 atm.
  s. Wires out: end result
  t. Wires out: end result

Marie-Claude Morice:

This is another type 4 lesion which does not involve the proximal segment and the diagonal branch originating proximal to the stenosis. I would have used the same treatment as in case 1, i.e. a short stent to the LAD with a protective wire in the diagonal. A similar phenomenon would probably have occurred: the plaque would have been shifted onto the diagonal ostium thus compromising the diagonal. I would have deployed a 3.0 mm balloon in the diagonal with simultaneous inflation of the 3.0 mm balloon in the stent to the LAD. In our experience, completing PTCA of a bifurcation with kissing inflation stabilizes the bifurcation and the plaque and prevents the 'snow-plough' phenomenon which frequently occurs when alternate dilatations are performed.

The final results achieved in this particular example are remarkable.

Antonio Colombo:

A 'Y' stent approach is described. This approach is also called the culottes technique. The best stents for this technique are CrossFlex™, CrossFlex LC™, MULTI-LINK®, DUET™, or TETRA™. In this particular example we would try to limit stenting to the major branch only. We reserve the 'Y' stent technique for situations in which we performed debulking on both branches or when the result following angioplasty on the side branch is grossly suboptimal.

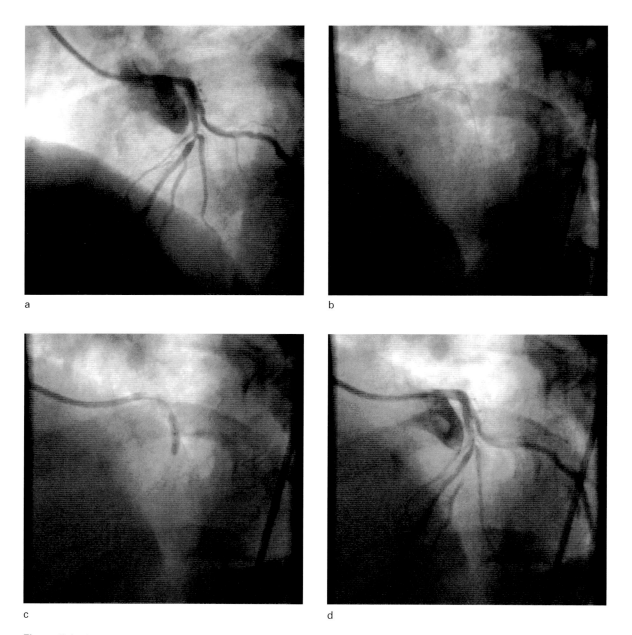

a

b

c

d

Figure 5.4a–t
a) Diagnostic in LAO cranial projection. b) 0.014" high torque floppy wires to both LAD and D1. c) 3.0 mm monorail balloon inflation in LAD lesion. d) Result of c.

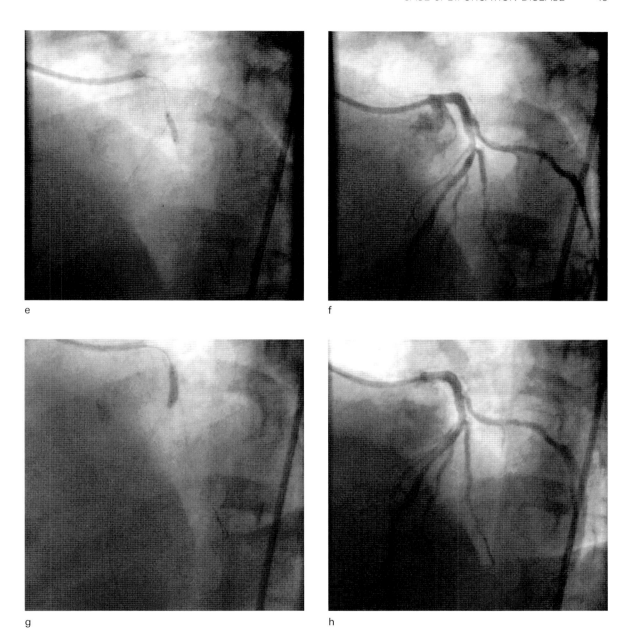

e

f

g

h

Figure 5.4 *continued*
e) 3.0 mm monorail balloon inflation in D1 lesion. f) Result of e. g) 3.0 mm × 15 mm Cordis CrossFlex™ stent in LAD across D1 origin. h) Result in LAO cranial view.

continued

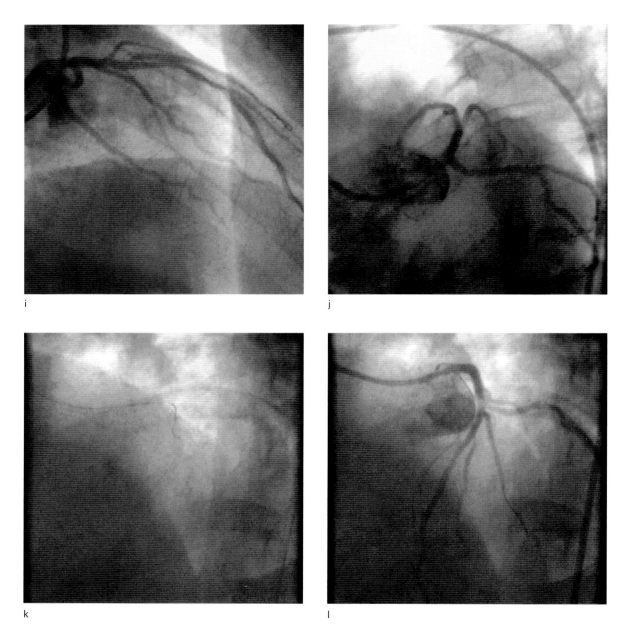

Figure 5.4 *continued*
i) Result in RAO view. j) Result in LAO caudal view. k) Pull back D1 wire into proximal LAD and then l) Pass it back into D1 through the side of the LAD stent.

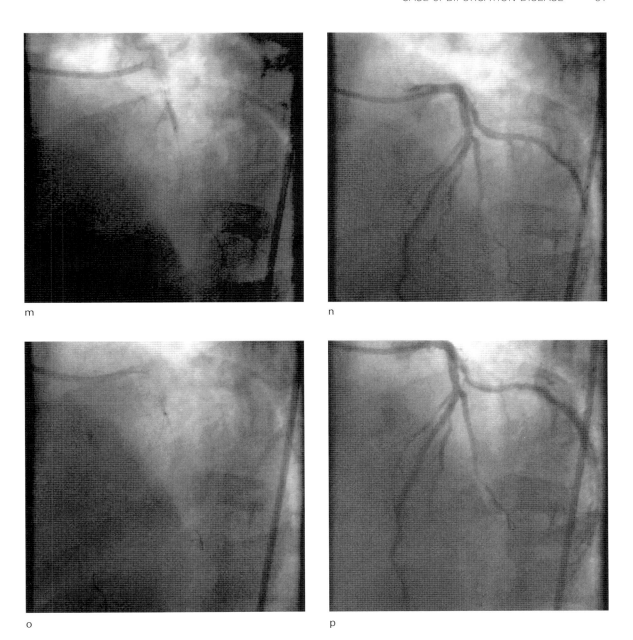

Figure 5.4 *continued*
m) 2.5 mm monorail balloon inflated through side of LAD stent to 12 atm. n) Result of m. o) Position Cordis CrossFlex™ 3.0 mm × 15 mm stent into D1 from LAD via the side of the LAD stent and pull back LAD wire before inflation. *p) Result.*

continued

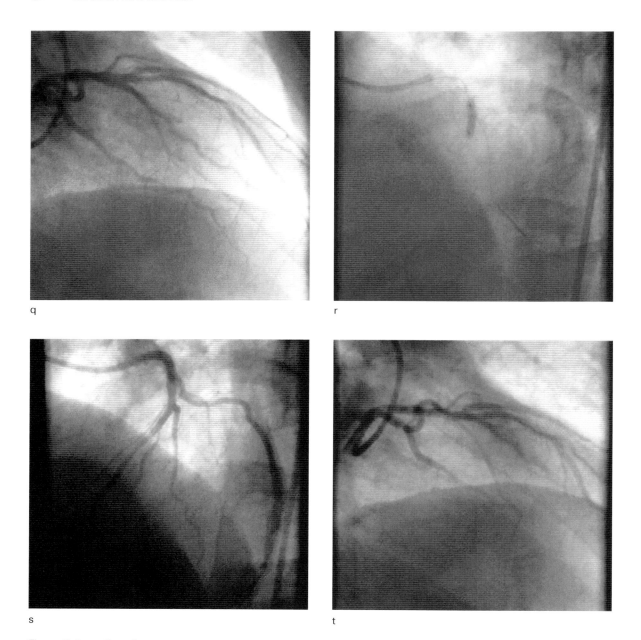

Figure 5.4 *continued*
q) Result. r) Pass LAD wire back down LAD through side of D1 stent, and then inflate 2.5 mm monorail balloon through side to 12 atm. s) Wires out: end result. t) Wires out: end result.

Case 4. Bifurcation disease

65-year-old man. Ex-smoker. Rapidly worsening angina.

Catheter findings: Well preserved LV function; tight stenosis in LAD involving origin of first diagonal branch; minor RCA disease.

Procedure: JL4 (8F) guide; 0.014″ high torque floppy wires to LAD and first diagonal (D1). Pre-dilatation of both vessels using a 3.0 mm monorail balloon. True 'Y' stent then fashioned using:

(a) 3.5 mm × 15 mm ACS MULTI-LINK® stent in LAD across diagonal origin;
(b) 3.0 mm × 15 mm ACS MULTI-LINK® stent into diagonal from LAD.

Both stents dilated with 3.5 mm Tacker balloon.

Marie-Claude Morice:

This is a type 1 LAD–diagonal bifurcation. The plaque involves the proximal and distal segments and stenosis is present in the diagonal. I would have selected type A treatment which involves insertion of a wire in each of the two branches, pre-dilatation followed by placement of a short 3.0 mm × 8.0 mm GFX stent in the diagonal, stenting of the LAD with a 15 mm beStent™ mounted on a 3.5 mm VIVA, with the diagonal wire jailed outside the proximal segment of the stent. After pulling back the wire from the diagonal and reinserting it inside both stents proximally and out into the diagonal distally I would have completed the procedure with a kissing balloon inflation (3.0 mm to diagonal and 3.5 mm to LAD) through a 6F JL4 guiding catheter. After several attempts on the test bench, we abandoned the crossed stent procedure (also called true 'Y' or culottes) because of poor results and too much metal at the bifurcation site. In this particular case, the diagonal branch being large and diseased, it should be stented first before a stent is placed in the LAD to avoid stenting through the struts of the LAD stent.

Editors: We share the concern about the long term results of the true 'Y' stent and await our outcome with interest.

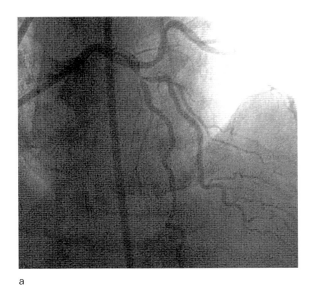

a

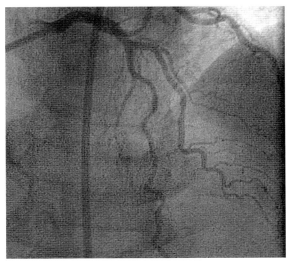

b

Figure 5.5
LCA angiogram. a) LAD/diagonal bifurcation stenosis. b) Result.

Antonio Colombo:

This is a bifurcation involving two large branches where both vessels could be dilated to 3.5 mm. The 'Y' stent or culottes technique appears appropriate, as is the use of the MULTI-LINK® or DUET™ stent. The large plaque mass in this bifurcation with significant involvement of both branches strongly points to the need to use a double stent approach. Even if technically more demanding, the 'Y' stent technique will give the best immediate results.

Our approach in this large plaque mass lesion is always to perform directional atherectomy on both branches and then proceed with 'Y' stenting.

A caveat concerning 'Y' stenting is to deploy the first stent always in the most angulated branch, which is usually the diagonal.

Case 5. Bifurcation disease

59-year-old man. Ex-smoker, NIDDM. CABG surgery 1987: vein grafts to LAD and OM of circumflex. Recurrent limiting angina.

Catheter findings: Moderate overall LV function; native LCA shows occluded LAD and significant circumflex and OM disease; OM vein graft occluded; LAD vein graft patent; RCA non-dominant.

Procedure: JL4 8F guide; 0.014″ high torque floppy wires to atrioventricular branch of the circumflex coronary artery (AVCx) and OM. 2.5 mm monorail balloon to both limbs and the stents:

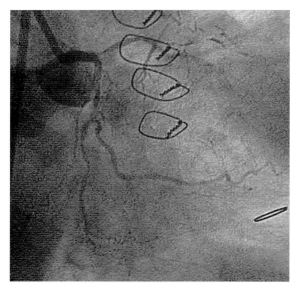
a

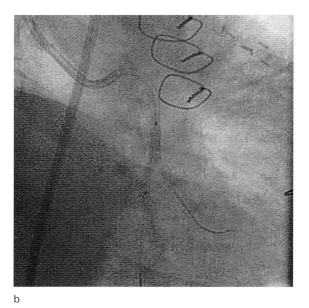
b

Figure 5.6a–e
LCA angiogram. a) Circumflex/OM bifurcation stenosis. b) Balloon dilatation of main Cx with side branch protection.

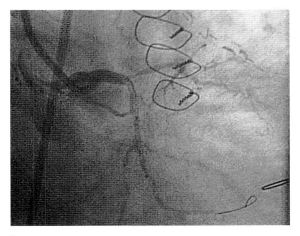

c

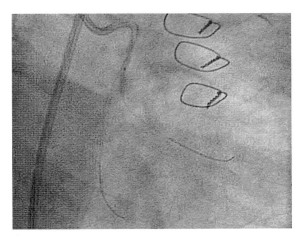

d

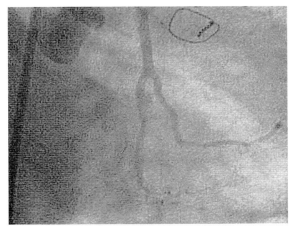

e

1. AVE GFX 3.0 mm × 18 mm in AVCx across OM origin
2. AVE GFX 3.0 mm × 18 mm into OM from AVCx
3. These two stents arranged as true 'Y' stent.
4. AVE GFX 3.5 mm × 24 mm from LMS into AVCx

Marie-Claude Morice:

This is a circumflex–marginal bifurcation with a long lesion involving the proximal segment of the circumflex. The distal segment of the circumflex does not seem significantly stenosed. It is a small vessel vascularizing a small territory and I would have avoided stenting it. I would have used two wires to protect the two branches. I would have dilated to the circumflex and the marginal with a 30 mm long 3.0 VIVA balloon in order to cover the whole lesion and then implanted a 25 mm beStent™ covering the circumflex and the marginal of the bifurcation to achieve optimal coverage. The guidewire to the distal circumflex would have been 'jailed' along side of the circumflex stent. We often perform such a procedure without cutting the wire (only when using an ACS wire).

The PT Graphic wires are very good wires but they should not be used in this particular case because they could easily break. If it had been necessary to dilate the distal circumflex after implantation of a stent in the proximal circumflex, we would have pulled back the wire from the distal circumflex, reinserted it with a 2.5 mm VIVA and performed kissing balloon inflation with a 3.0 mm VIVA in the marginal.

It is to be noted that the technique used by the operator led to an excellent result. There is more than one way to perform a procedure!

Antonio Colombo:

This is a bifurcation of a large obtuse marginal branch and a smaller posterolateral branch. The 'Y' technique used in this instance had produced an immediate favourable result. The usage of the GFX stent for this approach is very appropriate and most probably the simplest, besides the one

Figure 5.6 *continued*
c) Balloon dilatation of side branch with Cx protection. d) Proximal vessel dilatation. e) Result of true Y stenting and additional proximal stent.

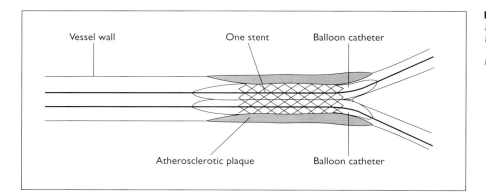

Figure 5.6f
Schematic description of the approach for a 'Pseudo-bifurcation' lesion

stent (in the major branch) technique. Our view is to stay more conservative with the usage of the 'Y' approach and reserve it for medium-sized vessels.

In this type of lesion, where the largest plaque mass is proximal to the bifurcation, we favour stent deployment proximally to the bifurcation and opening of the stent toward both branches with the one stent – two hugging balloon technique. This approach is outlined in the figures below.

Figure 5.6f shows the single stent hand mounted on two balloons. The distal ends of the balloons are located into the two branches, ensuring that the distal end of the stent is located at the carina of the bifurcation.

Figure 5.6g in the left panel shows the stent in situ in the coronary artery; the distal ends of the balloons can clearly be seen to be separated as they sit in the proximal portions of their respective vessels. The middle panels show each balloon opened separately toward its side

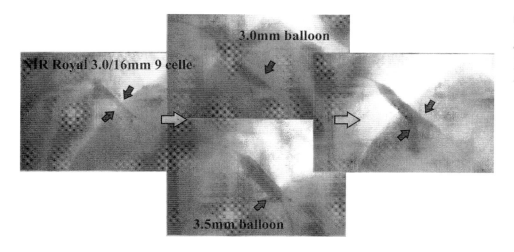

Figure 5.6g
Technique for pseudo-bifurcation lesion: 'Single stent with two balloons'

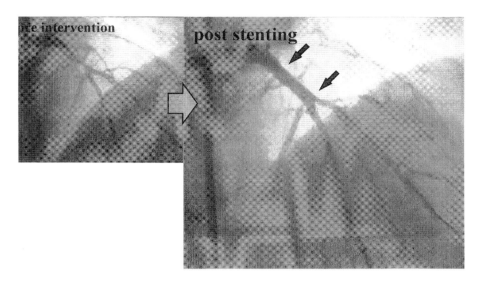

Figure 5.6h
*Result of 'single stent
with two balloons' for
'pseudo-bifurcation'
lesion*

branch. The right panel shows both balloons inflated to finish the procedure with the 'kissing balloon' technique.

Figure 5.6h illustrates an angiographic example of this technique.

The NIR™ Royal appears in our experience the best stent for this approach. We reserve this 'one stent – two hugging balloon' technique for lesions where the largest plaque mass is present proximal to the bifurcation and the origin of both branches creates a true 'Y' shape with an angle relatively narrow between the two branches.

Case 6. Bifurcation disease

54-year-old man. Hypertension. Limiting angina and early positive ETT.

Catheter findings: LV good; circumflex and RCA unobstructed; tight stenosis involving bifurcation of LAD and the first diagonal (D1).

Procedure: JL4 (8F); 0.014″ high torque floppy wires to LAD and D1. 3.0 mm monorail balloon to both. ACS MULTI-LINK® 3.0 mm × 20 mm in LAD; ACS MULTI-LINK® 3.0 mm × 25 mm to D1 as true 'Y' stent; Cordis CrossFlex™ 3.0 mm × 15 mm overlapping distal end of ACS MULTI-LINK® in D1.

Marie-Claude Morice:

This is apparently a type 2 lesion involving the LAD proximal and distal to a disease-free diagonal. I would have selected a type B treatment and inserted a wire in each branch, with subsequent pre-dilatation of both branches, placement of a tubular beStent™-type stent in the LAD, with the guidewire left in place in the diagonal. If deterioration of the diagonal ostium had occurred due to a 'snow-plough' phenomenon involving the LAD plaque, I would have withdrawn the wire from along side the beStent™, reinserted it through the side of the stent into the diagonal and performed a kissing balloon inflation (3.5 mm and 3.0 mm balloons) in both branches. If the diagonal ostium had remained stenosed and dissected, I would have implanted a short 3.0 mm GFX through the struts of the beStent™.

One may wonder why the wire should be left in place in the diagonal during placement of a stent in the LAD. The reason is that the wire keeps the branch open. In the case of a very deteriorated diagonal ostium, we generally pull back the LAD wire and reinsert it in parallel with the diagonal wire before removing the jailed wire and reinserting it in the LAD.

As mentioned earlier we always complete our procedure by a kissing balloon inflation in order to remodel the two stents. The technique of opening the struts of a stent to access a side branch causes a deformation of the opposite side of the stent. Kissing inflation restores the shape of the stent.

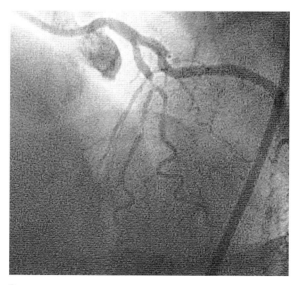

a

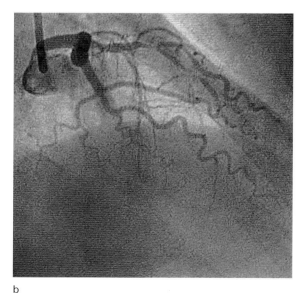

b

Figure 5.7a–f
LCA angiogram. a,b) LAD/diagonal stenosis.

Antonio Colombo:

This is another example involving the usage of the 'Y' technique. The same considerations expressed for case 4 apply to this case. In this situation we would be a little more conservative toward stenting both branches, owing to the medium size of the diagonal branch. If a double stenting approach needs to be used, the 'Y' is the most appropriate, because of the angle of origin (acute) of the diagonal from the LAD. Debulking with directional coronary atherectomy (DCA) and then stenting is another more demanding alternative.

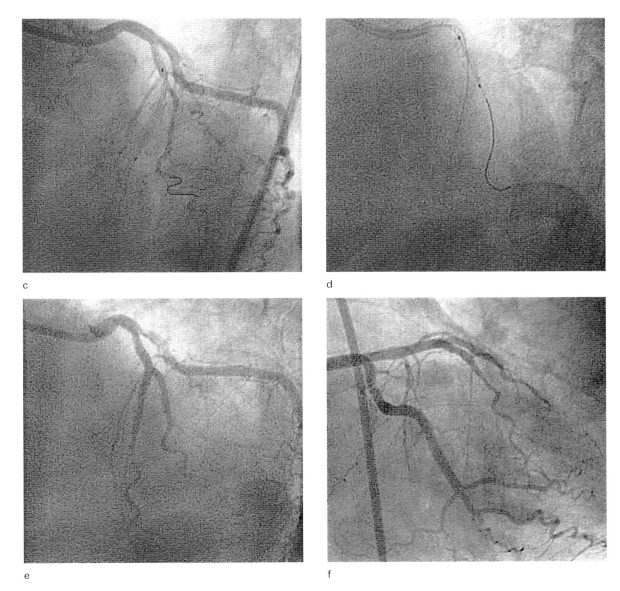

c

d

e

f

Figure 5.7 *continued*
c,d) Formation of 'Y' stent. e,f) Result.

Case 7. Bifurcation disease

69-year-old man. Hypertension; high cholesterol; ex-smoker. CABG surgery 1990: vein grafts to OM, LAD and RCA. Previous PTCA and stent to LAD vein graft. Stable angina and exercise test showed inferolateral ST depression.

Catheter findings: Poor LV function; occluded LAD, circumflex and RCA proximally; patent grafts to LAD and RCA; significant disease at distal anastomosis of vein graft both in antegrade direction (into OM) and retrogradely into AVCx via OM.

Procedure: Left graftseeker guide (8F); 0.014″ wires to both limbs. Pre-dilatation both ways with 3.0 mm monorail balloon, then true 'Y' fashioned using Cordis CrossFlex™ 3.0 mm × 25 mm stents in both directions.

Marie-Claude Morice:

According to our classification, this is a type 4, T-shaped lesion which is relatively easy to treat with a wire in each branch, simultaneous pre-dilatation of the two branches with a 3.0 mm

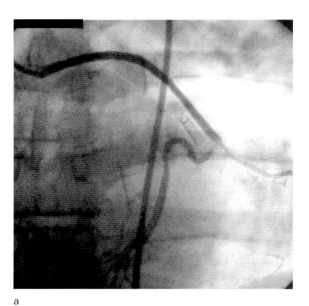

a

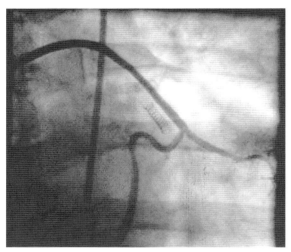

b

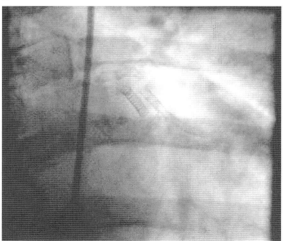

c

Figure 5.8
OM graft angiogram. a) Bifurcation disease at insertion site of graft, not stent in another vessel. b) Result. c) Non-contrasted image to show 'Y' stent.

VIVA balloon followed by implantation of two beStent™-type 15 mm stents or 8.0 mm stents delivered simultaneously through a 6F guide catheter.

Antonio Colombo:

The 'Y' technique can be used in almost any bifurcation where both branches are of appropriate size for stenting.

The most angulated branch should be stented first; a kissing inflation should always be performed at the very end of the procedure. This approach will minimize stent distortion, which invariably favours the last inflated stent. Ormistron et al. performed a detailed in-vitro evaluation of stent behaviour during the 'Y' stenting[4] and demonstrated the value of the kissing final inflation with the suggestion of first deflating the balloon located in the stent of the most angulated branch. This manoeuvre will prevent stent protrusion from the stent located in the side branch into the major branch.

Editors' summary

These cases illustrate the variety of different techniques and approaches available for treatment of bifurcation disease. Our view, shared by our experts, is that treatment should be tailored to the individual case. We are interested to see that Dr. Morice is comfortable with using two delivery systems through the 6F guide, including for kissing balloons, and we are fascinated by Dr Colombo's 'one stent–two hugging balloon' technique. Restenosis data are still sparse for the various bifurcation stenting techniques but current data suggest the restenosis rates for the 'Y' stent are high, particularly without the kissing technique.

References

1. Anzuini, et al. Wiktor stent for treatment of chronic total coronary artery occlusions; short and long-term clinical and angiographic results from a large multicenter experience. J Am Coll Cardiol 1998;31:281–288.
2. Carrie D, et al. Coronary stenting of bifurcation lesions using 'T' or 'Reverse Y' configuration with Wiktor stent. Am J Cardiol 1998;82:1418–1421.
3. Moussa et al. Stenting After Optimal Lesion Debulking (SOLD) Registry. Angiographic and clinical outcome. Circulation 1998;98:1604–1609.
4. Ormiston JA, et al. Stent distortion during simulate side-branch dilatation. J Am Coll Cardiol 1998;31(Suppl A):1005–1008.

6
Left main stem disease

Interventionalists are drawn to the treatment of left main stem disease in a similar manner to the attraction a naked flame has for a moth! The left main coronary has until relatively recently been considered a surgical bastion, except in the case of lesions protected by the presence of patent grafts. There is occasionally the opportunity to perform an angioplasty on a patient who presents with an acutely occluded left main stem, as in one of our examples below. Increasingly, however, cardiologists are taking on left main lesions that do not fall into either of these categories.

Summary of dilemmas

- Length of balloon and diameter: is the aim just to make way for a stent?
- Duration of inflations
- In unprotected cases should both LAD and circumflex be wired?
- Should we expect surgical cover, and if so should a theatre actually be waiting?
- Is an intra-aortic balloon pump advisable?
- Are there cases where some distal dissection in the LMS can be left without referral for surgery?
- Is the left main a site that is especially suited to debulking therapy?
- Is the threshold for using ReoPro® lower than for other lesions?

Comments on cases were obtained from **Stephen G Ellis**, **Samir Kapadia**, **Seung-Jung Park** and **Jean Fajadet**.

Case 1. Left main stem disease: protected

51-year-old man. High cholesterol; ex-smoker. CABG surgery 1986 (LIMA to LAD). Stable but limiting angina now.

Catheter findings: LV moderate; LIMA excellent; RCA dominant and unobstructed; LMS and proximal LCA as shown.

Procedure: Left Voda 3.5 (8F) guide; 0.014″ high torque floppy wire into circumflex; LMS dilated with 3.0 mm monorail balloon, then Medtronic Wiktor® 4.0 mm × 15 mm to 10 atm.

Stephen G Ellis and Samir Kapadia:

This patient has a bifurcation lesion stenosis of the distal left main trunk that is protected by a patent LIMA graft to LAD. The stenosis in mid-portion LAD restricts flow to proximal diagonal and septal perforators from the patent LIMA. The circumflex territory, however, is the major target for revascularization. This is a commonly encountered anatomy in patients after bypass surgery. A functional assessment to localize ischaemia and scar can help to decide the relative importance of proximal LAD stenosis. In this young patient, considering these angiographic findings, it seems important to treat the proximal LAD to improve flow to the diagonal and septal perforators.

In this situation, rotational atherectomy of the distal LM trunk and LAD ostium followed by the same for the ostium of the circumflex can be helpful. The role of debulking with rotational atherectomy is not proven in LM lesions, however, it may be useful in this type of bifurcation lesion or in calcified vessels.[1] Treatment of the proximal LAD stenosis with balloon angioplasty along with rotational atherectomy may prove to be adequate. The most distal LAD stenosis should be left to protect the patency of the LIMA graft. In that case, stenting of the circumflex ostium, as done here, might be sufficient. The selection of the stent is dependent on the ease and feasibility of accessing the side branch (LAD) through the stent strut. However, given the presence of a patent and

Figure 6.1
LCA angiogram. a) Stenosis at the distal left main stem. b) Guidewires to LAD and Cx with balloon inflation in Cx origin. c) Final result.

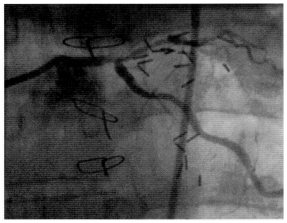

a

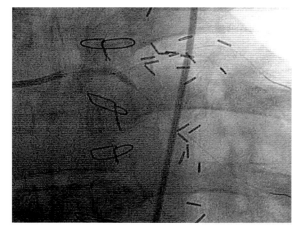

b

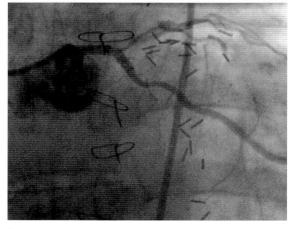

c

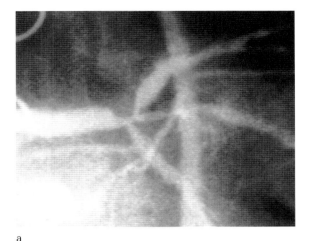

a

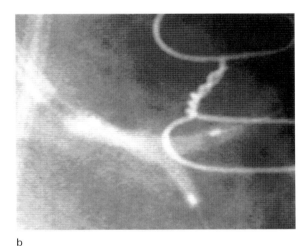

b

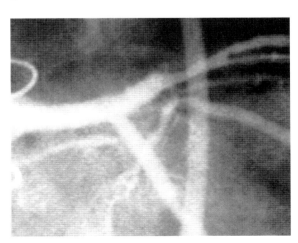

c

probably long-lived graft to the LAD, the treatment of distal LM trunk/ostial circumflex should not be compromised by the choice of a suboptimal stent. In this regard, we believe the Wiktor® is a poor choice. A DUET™, NIR™ (or NIR-side) or Crown can give a better long-term result.

An alternative would be to perform 'T' stenting after kissing balloon angioplasty. The case from our centre (Fig. 6.2a–c) demonstrates this point. This is a patient with a distal LM trunk lesion and a protected ramus intermedius and LAD with a small left circumflex coronary artery (LCX). Two wires were placed in LAD and circumflex and lesions individually dilated. A stent was passed beyond the LAD ostium and then another stent was placed in the LCX. After placing the stent as close to the ostium of the LCX as possible the LAD stent was pulled back to ascertain the position of the proximal end of the LCX stent at the ostium and not in the LM trunk. The LCX stent was then deployed and the LAD stent was then appropriately placed to cover the distal LM trunk and LAD ostium and then deployed. This approach has been limited by a heightened risk of restenosis, however. That debulking prior to stenting would decrease this risk is suspected but not proven.[2]

Seung-Jung Park:

The patency of a grafted vessel to the left coronary artery system is very important. The LIMA supplies coronary flow to the LAD in this case. Therefore, even though it is a left main lesion, in practical terms it is safe to consider it as single vessel disease in the proximal portion of the left circumflex artery.

Stent selection in this case does not seem to be an issue; for it does not involve the ostium of the left main coronary artery: either a slotted tube stent or coil stent would do the job. In terms of acute stent recoil, stents such as the Wiktor® and the Tantalum Cordis have a higher acute stent recoil immediately after stent deployment. Recently developed coil stents such as the CrossFlex™ and GFX have comparable radial forces to those of slotted tube stents so can be considered for this application.

Figure 6.2
LCA angiogram. a) Distal LM stenosis involving LAD and Cx. b) Simultaneous dilatation of kissing balloons. c) Result.

Case 2. Left main stem disease: unprotected

56-year-old man. Ex-smoker, high cholesterol. Starr–Edwards aortic valve replacement for aortic stenosis September 1996. Acute infective endocarditis with valve dehiscence leading to emergency replacement of aortic valve with further Starr–Edwards February 1999. Postoperatively required permanent pacemaker. Developed limiting exertional angina April 1997.

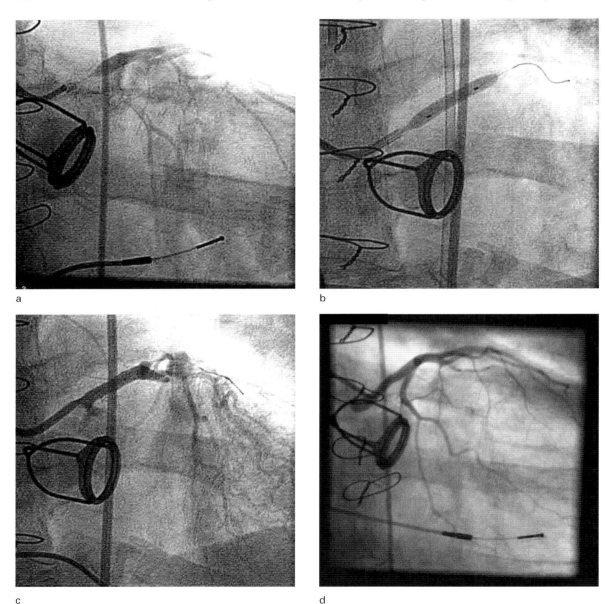

a

b

c

d

Figure 6.3
LCA angiogram. a) Proximal LM disease. b) Stent deployment, guide catheter displaced. c) Immediate result. d) 6 months follow-up.

Thallium scan showed extensive area of reversible ischaemia.

Catheter findings: right left main stem stenosis with remaining coronaries unobstructed.

Procedure: JL4; 0.014″ high torque floppy wire. 3.0 mm monorail balloon. 4.0 mm × 15 mm ACS MULTI-LINK® stent.
Abciximab (ReoPro®).

Follow-up: 6 month angiogram (Fig. 6.3d)

Stephen G Ellis and Samir Kapadia:

This patient has unprotected left main trunk (ULMT) ostial stenosis with an unobstructed dominant RCA. The patient already had open-heart surgery twice and has a well functioning aortic valve. He can be treated with percutaneous intervention although angiographic follow-up is advisable within 6–8 weeks.

Stenting of the unprotected LMT was associated with a better outcome in hospital than balloon angioplasty alone, in the ULTIMA registry, the largest series of ULMT interventions.[3] Therefore, balloon dilatation using a relatively small balloon is appropriate for pre-dilatation prior to stenting. Short balloon inflations of 15–30 seconds as tolerated by the patient can be used. A stent with good radial strength as used in this patient is appropriate. The role of debulking is unsettled but this can be considered in stable patients with severely calcified vessels, especially if they have normal left ventricular systolic function.

The support devices such as IABP and CPS have been used to different extents in previously published series.[3,4] Their utilization is predominantly determined by patient characteristics. IABP or CPS should be considered in patients with poor left ventricular function, unstable symptoms, dominant LCX or compromised dominant RCA. Assuming a normally functioning prosthetic aortic valve and LV function, the experienced unprotected LMT operator will probably be able to do without IABP or CPS. An IABP should be placed if the operator is concerned that it might be needed.

Surgical backup is beneficial but not essential as most of the patients who undergo LMT stenting are either not candidates for surgery, or surgery is impractical due to severe comorbidity limiting life expectancy.

Percutaneous intervention is still not recommended in the patients who are good surgical candidates, as there is an early, unexplained mortality risk with percutaneous intervention.[3] Considering the recent data to show short- and long-term benefit with abciximab prior to percutaneous intervention, its use is appropriate in this case.

Seung-Jung Park

The most important thing to consider in performing unprotected left main stenting is the safety related to a left ventricular function. If the patient has good left ventricular function, then haemodynamic support (IABP) may not be really necessary.

Usually the balloon inflation takes only 10–20 seconds and it is therefore so brief that haemodynamic derangement does not take place. When the ostium of the left main coronary artery is involved, a slotted tube stent is preferable over a coil stent to provide sufficient support to deliver relatively high radial force. Also, the diameter of the stent should be approximately 0.5 mm larger than the reference vessel diameter. Then the stent is deployed for 10–15 seconds by the single high-pressure inflation method.

In our practice unprotected left main stenting is generally accompanied by IVUS evaluation so that we can be assured of stent apposition.

In the Asian Medical Centre more than 100 unprotected left main stenting procedures have been performed. However since none of the patients had poor left ventricular function, we have not used IABP or other forms of LV support technology thus far.

Case 3. Left main stem disease

72-year-old woman. Ex-smoker; high cholesterol; diabetes. Jehovah's Witness. Limiting exertional angina.

Catheter findings: Significant LAD and RCA disease with moderate LV.

Procedure:
LAD: JL4; 0.014″ high torque floppy wire. Pre-dilatation with 3.0 mm monorail balloon. Overlapping stent from distal to proximal: (a) Cordis CrossFlex™ 3.0 mm × 25 mm; (b) Cordis CrossFlex™ 3.0 mm × 15 mm.
RCA: JR4; 0.014″ high torque floppy wire. Pre-dilatation with 3.0 mm monorail balloon, then Jomed 3.0 mm × 16 mm stent.

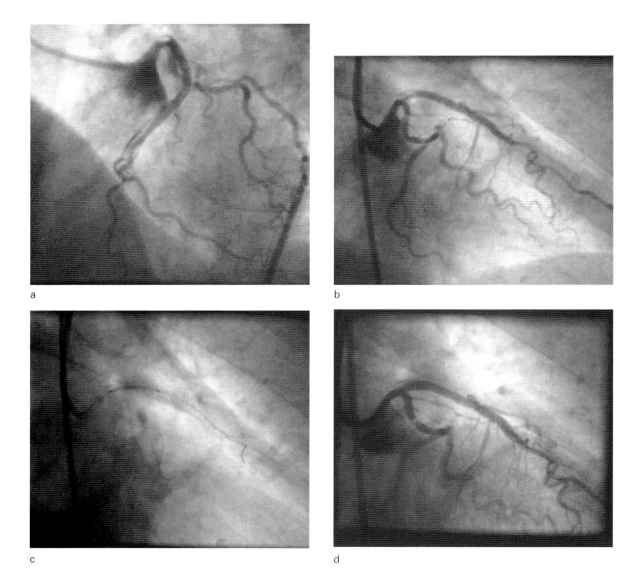

a   b

c   d

Figure 6.4a–d
LCA angiogram. a) Dissection proximally, LAD or LM? b) RAO view confirming ostial LAD dissection extending back to LM. c) Stent to ostial LAD. d) Result.

60 minutes after leaving the laboratory, the patient developed widespread inferior ST elevation followed a few minutes later by chest pain. RCA showed stent thrombosis. Abciximab (ReoPro®) given and RCA opened with 3.0 mm monorail balloon. Distally there was haziness, and a further stent (Cordis CrossFlex™ 3.0 mm × 15 mm) was deployed overlapping the distal end of the first stent with a good result. Diagnostic pictures of the left demonstrated a dissection in the LMS, as shown. The patient refused theatre (abciximab [ReoPro®] on board and Jehovah's Witness!). Therefore, a Cordis CrossFlex™ 3.5 mm × 15 mm stent was deployed from the proximal LAD back to the junction with the LMS. Uneventful recovery.

Stephen G Ellis and Samir Kapadia:

This is an unfortunate patient with dissection of the unprotected LM trunk where surgery is not an option. Abciximab was given for the treatment of RCA, but it would have been a reasonable adjuvant treatment for this type of dissection in itself.

In this patient, the extent of the dissection in relation to the coronary ostia should be precisely delineated. Intravascular ultrasound may help to accomplish this if the patient is haemodynamically stable. If the dissection extends well into the LM trunk and the circumflex ostium is not diseased, as in this case, the entire dissection should be covered with a stent. A stent that allows easy access to a side branch yet resists restenosis should be used, as we discussed in our comments to case 1. This will jail the ostium of the circumflex but should not compromise flow. However, plaque shifting to compromise the circumflex ostium has been well described in this setting. If the ostium of the circumflex is involved in the dissection, one should consider wiring both vessels and possibly using 'T' or 'Y' stenting. The circumflex may also need to be wired and treated if the ostium is significantly diseased or it is moderately diseased but has an unfavourable angle for wiring. Verifying the final results of the intervention with intravascular ultrasound in this case can be helpful.

Seung-Jung Park:

Both to examine the dissection clearly and to delineate lesion characteristics effectively I would recommend IVUS evaluation.

If the dissection extends from the proximal LAD to the distal left main coronary artery and it is a pure dissection then the deployment of the Cordis CrossFlex™ stent seems quite reasonable.

If there is no evidence of disease in the ostium of the left circumflex artery, even though stent jail will occur, long-term patency is relatively high (unpublished data). In addition, if the left circumflex artery is not a dominant system it seems safe to deploy a stent down to the distal portion of left main coronary artery.

If there were significant disease in the ostium of the left circumflex coronary artery then the protection of the left circumflex artery with a guidewire would be the first thing required. After the dissection is treated then a second intervention such as balloon dilatation and/or another stent deployment could be performed in the left circumflex artery through the stent struts. In this way surgery may be avoided.

The final angiogram in this case showed that the whole dissection was not covered with the CrossFlex™ stent.

I would recommend IVUS evaluation of this kind of dissection after stenting.[4]

In our centre we have performed a number of procedures employing debulking prior to stent implantation and a case example is provided below (Fig. 6.5e,f).

These angiograms show highly significant distal LM disease (Fig. 6.5g,h).

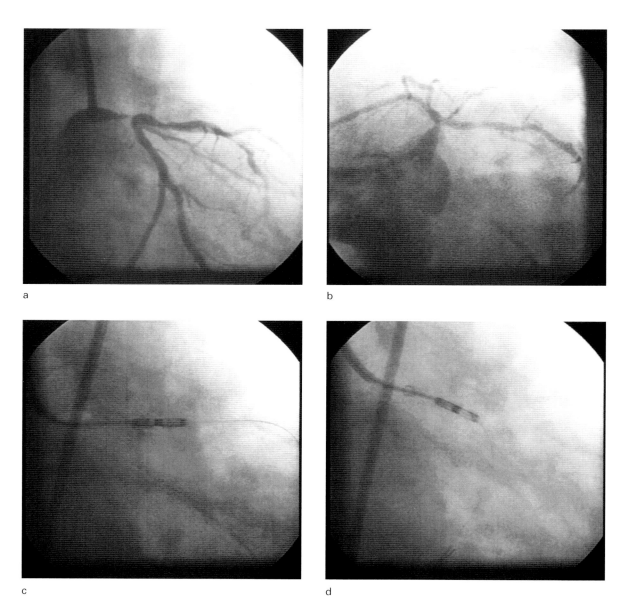

a

b

c

d

Figure 6.5a–f
LCA angiogram. a) Distal LM stenosis. b) Atherectomy of LM/LAD junction. c) Spider-view to show initial result. d) Atherectomy of LM/Cx.

Directional atherectomy was undertaken into the LAD and then into the circumflex coronary arteries (Fig. 6.5e,f). Note that only one guidewire is used during this portion of the procedure.

The angiograms show the excellent result obtained after debulking and stenting of the LM.

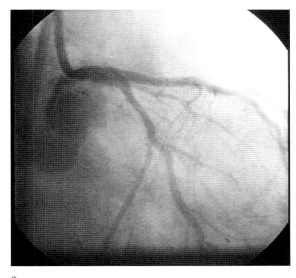

e

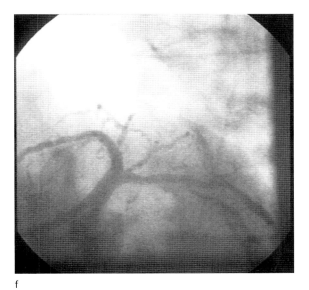

f

Figure 6.5 *continued*
e,f) Final result.

Jean Fajadet provides the following cases for discussion

Case 4. Unprotected left mainstem disease

84-year-old man. Unstable angina.

Catheter findings: Good LV with left ventricular ejection fraction (LVEF) = 60%; severe 80% stenosis distal left main trunk; LAD, circumflex coronary artery (CX) and RCA unobstructed; Qualitative coronary angiography (QCA) on-line showed 81% stenosis of the distal left main; reference diameter 3.1 mm.
There was no evidence of heavy calcification on fluoroscopy.

Procedure: We used the transradial approach with a 6F guiding catheter with a 6F sheath.
Guiding catheter: JL3.5 Extra Back-up 6F Cordis Vista Brite Tip™ catheter with inner lumen of 0.64″. Guidewire: 0.014″ BMW (ACS).
The balloon was inflated without any previous debulking procedure. Balloon catheter: 3.0 mm Bonnie™ balloon (Schneider).
The stent used was the Cordis CrossFlex™: 3.0 × 15 mm.

Jean Fajadet:

In this 84-year-old man we used the transradial approach in order to reduce the risk of vascular access site complications. The distal LM stenosis is seen in Fig. 6.6a of case 4. The reference diameter of the left main was 3.1 mm (Fig. 6.6b) so we used a 6F guide catheter which allows access for 3.0 mm or 3.5 mm stents.

In the absence of heavy calcification on fluoroscopy we are happy to perform balloon dilatation without a debulking procedure. We only use the Rotablator when fluoroscopy shows the presence of calcification.

The balloon was inflated three times for 30 seconds at high pressure up to 18 atm (Fig. 6.4c). The angiographic result after this showed a good dilatation of the narrowing but with a 30% of residual stenosis (Fig. 6.6d). Angioplasty was therefore completed with a CrossFlex™ stent implantation, with the device deployed at 18 atm with an excellent angiographic result (Figs. 6.6e–g).

It is important to note that the origin of the circumflex artery remains widely patent after stent implantation with no encroachment of the device so that a protective guidewire was not employed.

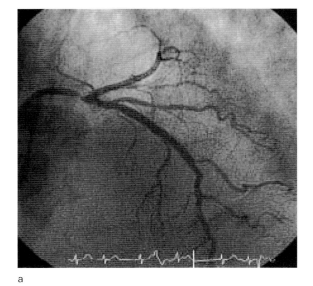

a

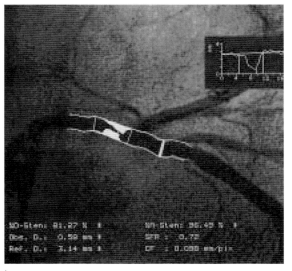

b

Figure 6.6a–g
LCA angiogram. a) Distal LM stenosis. b) QCA result.

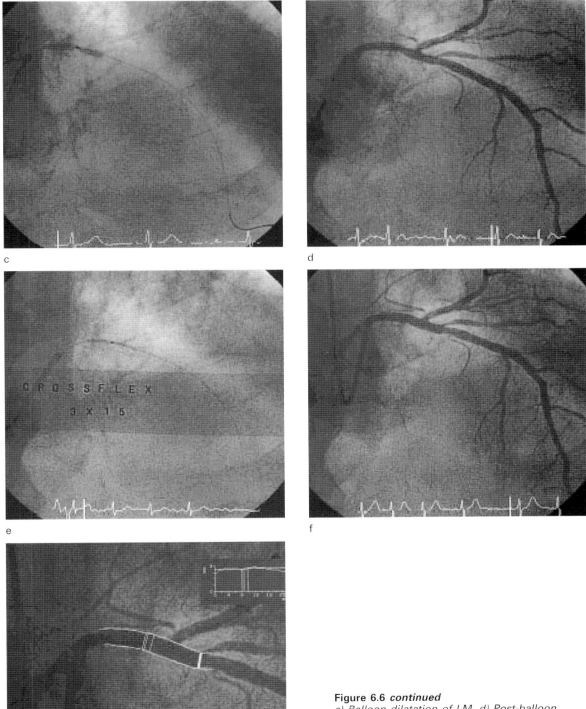

Figure 6.6 *continued*
c) Balloon dilatation of LM. d) Post-balloon dilatation. e) Stent placement. f) Result after stent. g) QCA result.

Case 5. Unprotected left mainstem disease

76-year-old man. Recent non-Q MI; hypertension, chronic bronchopneumonia, myopathy, abdominal aortic aneurysm and history of TIAs.

Catheter findings: Impaired LV with LVEF = 40%; severe stenosis of distal left main trunk; LAD, CX and RCA without significant disease.
QCA on-line showed the MLD of the distal left main to be 1.5 mm; reference diameter 4.1 mm.

Procedure: We used the transradial approach with a 7F guiding catheter with a 7F sheath.

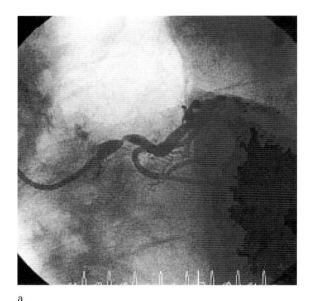

a

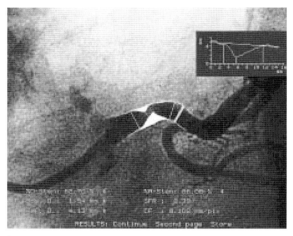

b

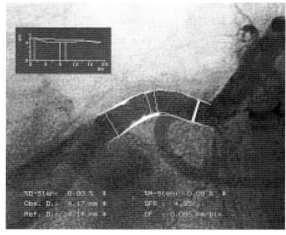

d

Figure 6.7
LCA angiogram. a) Mid-LM tight stenosis. b) QCA pre-dilatation. c) Result after stent. d) QCA result.

c

Guiding catheter: JL3.5 Extra back-up 7F Cordis Vista Brite Tip™ catheter with inner lumen of 0.64". Guidewire: 0.014" BMW (ACS).
The balloon catheter was 3.0 mm × 20 mm VIVA (Scimed) inflated for 10 seconds to 18 atm.
The stent used was the Cordis CrossFlex™: 4.0 mm × 15 mm inflated to 16 atm for 20 seconds and 15 seconds to give a final diameter of 4.3 mm.

Jean Fajadet:

This patient was unsuitable for CABG owing to concomitant illnesses. The radial approach was used to avoid the abdominal aortic aneurysm. The pre-procedure angiogram is seen in Fig. 6.5a. Note the good guide catheter position. The QCA prior to dilatation is seen in Fig. 6.7b.

A short inflation at high pressure was undertaken to create a passage for the stent. No blood pressure drop was noted. Likewise the stent was deployed with short high-pressure inflations. The post-stent angiogram is seen in Fig. 6.7c and the QCA in Fig. 6.7d.

We believe the CrossFlex™ coil stent has great adaptability and conforms to the vessel anatomy perfectly, the stent has high radial force.

At our centre the acute and mid-term (6–8 months) clinical results of stenting unprotected left main stenosis have been satisfactory, considering the severity of the pathology and the complicated clinical status (mainly old age) of these patients.

References

1. Ellis SG, Popma JJ, Buchbinder M, et al. Relation of clinical presentation, stenosis morphology, and operator technique to the procedural results of rotational atherectomy and rotational atherectomy-facilitated angioplasty. Circulation 1994;89: 882–892.
2. Moussa I, Moses J, Di Mario C, et al. Stenting After Optimal Lesion Debulking (SOLD) Registry. Angiographic and clinical outcome. Circulation 1998;98:1604–1609.
3. Ellis SG, Tamai H, Nobuyoshi M, et al. Contemporary percutaneous treatment of unprotected left main coronary stenoses: initial results from a multicenter registry analysis 1994–1996. Circulation 1997;96:3867–3872.
4. Park SJ, Park SW, Hong MK, et al. Stenting of unprotected left main coronary artery stenoses: immediate and late outcomes. J Am Coll Cardiol 1998;31:37–42.

7
Graft disease

Percutaneous revascularization of grafts provides the interventionist with a very diverse range of technical challenges. Perhaps because of the propensity for vein grafts to develop friable atheromatous material and thrombus, even the most apparently straightforward case carries with it the risk of sudden loss of flow due to distal embolization. Such considerations have led to a keen interest into methods for minimizing this, such as direct stenting, and devices for intercepting emboli before they reach the distal coronary. Recently occluded grafts containing a large burden of thrombus can be especially difficult to clear efficiently. Grafts are often performed upon patients who are at higher than average risk for major complications. Extensive areas of disease are often involved, prompting questions about the optimum length to cover with stent and whether some types of stent are especially suitable. The longer term outcome of stented grafts is also less clear than for native vessels.

Another area of technical challenge is the stenting of a native coronary via a graft, perhaps the ultimate example being the LAD via a LIMA graft. Finally, increasingly we are being presented with grafts whose access may be difficult or unusual.

In this chapter we present a range of graft cases with which we aim to explore these technical challenges.

Comments have been obtained from **Christopher J White, Christian W Hamm, Stephan Baldus, Christopher SR Baker** and **Martin T Rothman.**

Case 1. Grafts

54-year-old man. Hypertension; family history; hypercholesterolaemia. Presented with limiting exertional angina. 1984 CABG (vein grafts to LAD, OM, and RCA).

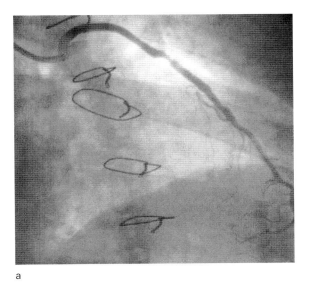

a

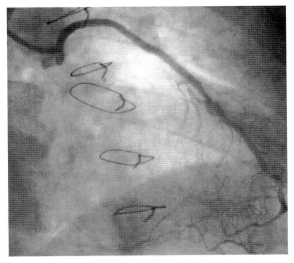

b

Figure 7.1
LAD graft angiogram. a) Mid-graft stenosis. b) Result.

Catheter findings: Good LV; occluded RCA; significant LMS and proximal LAD disease; vein graft to LAD 80% mid vessel stenosis; occluded VGs to OM and RCA.

Procedure: Left graftseeker (8F) guide; 0.014″ high torque floppy wire. Pre-dilatation with 3.0 mm monorail balloon. Segment stented with ACS MULTI-LINK® 3.5 mm × 25 mm to 12 atm.

Christopher J White:

I think that serious consideration should have been given to performing redo CABG with arterial conduits in this relatively young man with preserved LV function. Even after successful SVG–LAD intervention he will have continued ischaemia of the inferior wall, and with such old grafts the likelihood of failure due to either in-stent restenosis or the development of a new lesion is more than 50% at 1 year. Repeat bypass offers him the best chance of 'complete' revascularization and sustained clinical improvement.

In selecting a guiding catheter for a cranially oriented take-off of a vein graft, I would prefer an Amplatz shape, perhaps AL1 or AL1.5 or a 'hockeystick', which would allow a more coaxial alignment of the guiding catheter and ostium of the graft. I prefer an 8F guide when delivering 'Palmaz' biliary stents to vein grafts, but I prefer a large lumen (> 0.66″) 6F guiding catheter to deliver coronary stents.

I have a general preference for 'stiffer' extra support-type guidewires, which I believe aid delivery and trackability of stents into vein grafts. When using low profile coronary stents in lesions such as this, it is appropriate to attempt avoidance of pre-dilatation to minimize the risk of distal embolization during withdrawal.

I prefer to use longer, rather than shorter stents for vein graft disease. We know from IVUS and angioscopic imaging that the vein graft is diffusely diseased which makes complete coverage of the lesion the goal. The frequent occurrence of 'new' lesions during follow-up of vein graft stents supports the strategy of complete coverage rather than 'spot' stenting.

Case 2. Grafts

48-year-old man. Hypercholesterolaemia. CABG surgery 1988 (VGs to RCA and OM, LIMA to LAD). Limiting exertional angina.

Catheter findings: LV good; LAD occluded proximally; circumflex occluded proximally; severe native RCA disease; VG to RCA patent with good run off; LIMA to LAD patent with good run off; I stump; VG to OM as shown.

Procedure: Left graftseeker guide (8F); 0.014″ high torque floppy wire. 4.0 mm monorail balloon followed by NIR 4.0 mm × 16 mm stent mounted on a 5.0 mm ByPass Speedy balloon deployed at 12 atm.

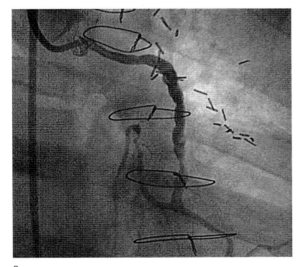

a

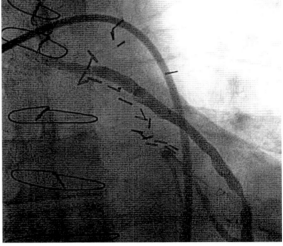

b

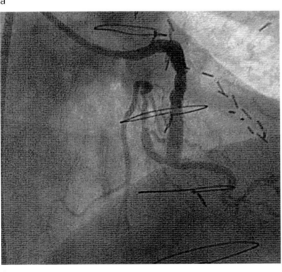

c

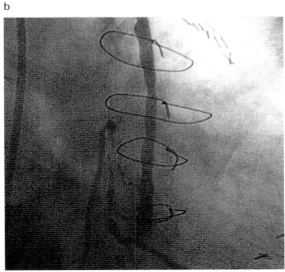

d

Figure 7.2
OM graft angiogram. a,b) Distal stenosis. c,d) Result.

Christopher J White:

I would consider using a Palmaz 'biliary' stent in this lesion instead of expanding a coronary stent to its upper limits. I would not favour graft reconstruction with a Wallstent® in this diffuse non-obstructive disease until there are convincing data that there is a true benefit.

Prevention of distal emboli is a challenging problem. I treat most vein graft lesions with abciximab (Reopro®) which does not prevent emboli from occurring but may minimize the sequelae of prolonged no-reflow. I avoid excessively high (> 12 atm) balloon inflation pressures in vein grafts to minimize distal emboli. We are currently gaining experience with the Percusurge device (Fig. 7.3a), which blocks run-off of embolic material with a distal occlusion balloon and then allows aspiration and removal of the material. The left panel shows the baseline angiogram with a tight proximal stenosis in the body of a vein graft, the middle panel shows the Percusurge balloon inflated (arrows). Aspiration of debris proximal to the balloon can take place through the catheter. The right panel shows the final result after stent placement and removal of the Percusurge catheter.

The distal location of the lesion in case 2 would make positioning and inflating of the Percusurge occlusion balloon difficult, and may well preclude its use in this case.

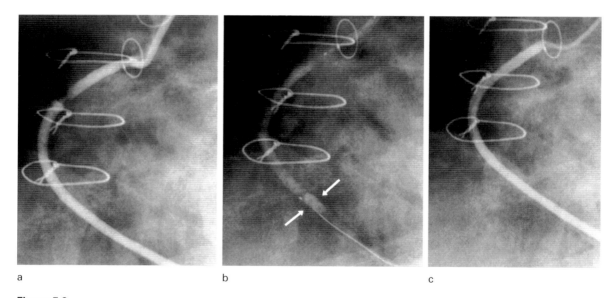

a   b   c

Figure 7.3
RCA angiogram. a) Lesion in proximal RCA. b) Distal position of Percusurge balloon seen at arrows. c) Result.

Case 3. Grafts

68-year-old man. Ex-smoker; high cholesterol. CABG surgery 8 years earlier: jump graft from diagonal to LAD; vein graft to RCA.
Stable angina.

Catheter findings: Moderate LV; patent vein grafts but lesion in LAD beyond insertion.

Procedure: Left graftseeker guide (8F); 0.014" high torque floppy wire; 2.5 mm Bypass Speedy balloon. Cordis CrossFlex™ 3.0 mm × 15 mm stent.

Christopher J White

With the small size of the native LAD (< 2.5 mm), I would try to avoid placing a stent. If it becomes necessary to stent a 2.5 mm vessel, I prefer slotted tubular stents which generally have a lower profile than coil stents, and in smaller vessels yield a larger post-stent MLD owing to less recoil. I prefer a stiffer-bodied guidewire to aid trackability of the balloons and stent to these distal lesions. Alternatively, a balloon-on-a-wire system, such as the ACE (Scimed) balloon, works very well in these potentially difficult to reach lesions.

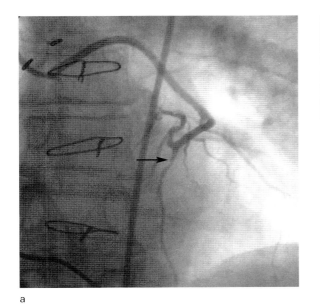
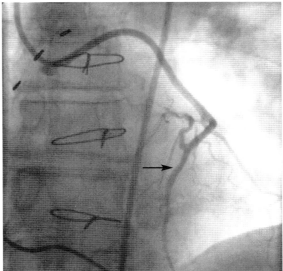

a

b

Figure 7.4
LAD graft angiogram. a) Lesion in native LAD. b) Result.

Case 4. Grafts

65-year-old man. Ex-smoker; hypertension. CABG surgery 1991 (vein grafts to LAD and RCA). Recurrent stable angina.

Catheter findings: Well preserved LV function; both grafts patent, but occlusion of native LAD beyond anastomosis.

Procedure: JR4 8F guide; 0.014" high torque floppy wire backed-up with 1.5 mm over-the-wire balloon for disobliteration, then 2.5 mm monorail balloon. Not stented.

Christopher J White:

My initial wire selection would have been an exchange length extra-support guidewire to facil-itate potential stent placement. If that failed to cross, my second choice would be a coated wire such as the Choice-PT™ (Scimed) or Crosswire™ (Cordis) also using an over-the-wire balloon for support. I would favour a 6F guiding catheter unless rotational atherectomy was being consid-ered, although the 1.5 mm burr may be used in a large-lumen (> 0.66") guiding catheter.

The best current evidence demonstrates a superior outcome when total occlusions are treated with stents.[1] The limitation in this case is the size of the target artery. I would have tried very hard to place a 3 mm balloon-expandable stent in this lesion. If, at the beginning of the procedure, I felt the vessel was too small to stent, I would strongly consider using rotational atherectomy to 'debulk' the total occlusion as an adjunct to balloon dilatation. While the angiographic appear-ance of the result obtained with balloon alone in this case is excellent, this is the exception rather than the rule in treating total occlusions.

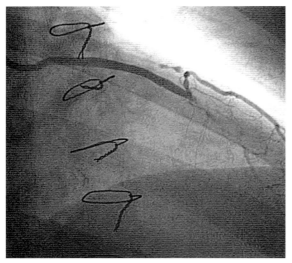

a

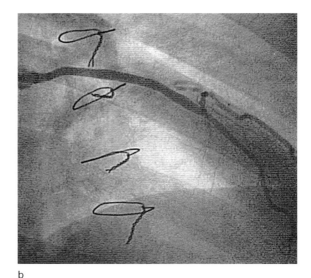

b

Figure 7.5
LAD angiogram. a) Total occlusion of native vessel. b) Result.

Case 5. Grafts

58-year-old man. Ex-smoker; hypertension. CABG 1987: vein grafts to LAD, OM, and RCA. Recurrent symptoms and investigation at a different hospital led to referral for redo CABG. Presented with unstable angina with anterior T wave changes and lateral ST depression.

Catheter findings: Occluded LMS; dominant RCA with tight distal stenosis; VG to LAD occluded with thrombus; vein graft to OM contained significant ostial and mid-vessel stenoses; VG to RCA had significant stenosis distally. LV moderate.

Procedure:
- LAD vein graft: left graftseeker 8F guide; 0.014″ high torque floppy wire. Multiple inflations along graft and at anastomosis with 3.0 mm monorail balloon. Three stents: distally 3.5 mm × 28 mm Guidant Duet at anastomosis overlapped in graft by Guidant Duet 4.0 mm × 23 mm. From ostium into graft a Guidant Duet 4.0 mm × 28 mm stent was deployed, crossing the line of occlusion.
- OM vein graft: left graftseeker 8F guide; 0.014″ high torque floppy wire. Pre-dilatation of mid-vessel stenosis with 3.5 mm monorail balloon followed by 4.0 mm × 28 mm Guidant Duet stent. More proximal lesion directly stented using Guidant Duet 4.0 mm × 23 mm.
- RCA VG: Amplatz Left Guide (8F); 0.014″ high torque floppy wire. Direct stent with 3.5 mm × 13 mm Guidant Duet.

Abciximab (ReoPro®).

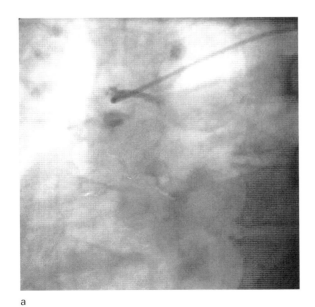

a

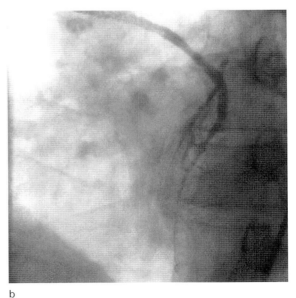

b

Figure 7.6a–g
a) Total occlusion of proximal LAD graft. b) Result of disobliteration and distal stent.

continued

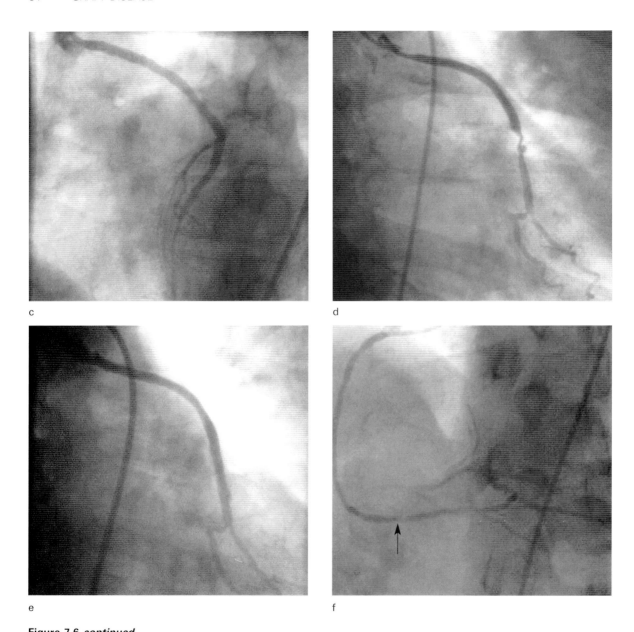

Figure 7.6 *continued*
c) Result of LAD graft. d) Ostial and mid-graft disease. e) Result of proximal and mid-graft stenting. f) RCA graft lesion (arrow).

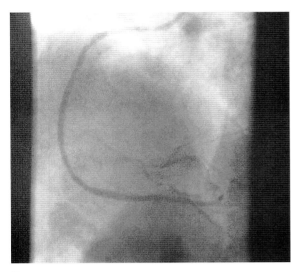

g

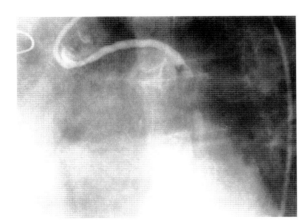

*

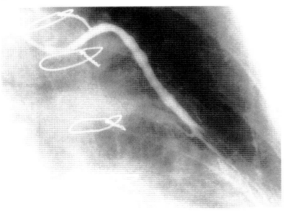

**

Christopher J White:

Intervention for acute coronary ischaemia is appropriate in this case, although in this relatively young man with 12-year-old vein grafts, redo bypass surgery with arterial conduits would have the advantage of greater durability than can be achieved with percutaneous intervention in degenerated vein grafts.

I agree with the strategy of treating multiple vessels at one sitting: as long as each result is excellent, I would not hesitate to continue on to the next vessel. For thrombosed vein grafts, particularly those with a large thrombus burden, my approach is to use aspiration thrombectomy with the Angiojet™ (Possis; Figs 7.6*,**) followed by balloon dilatation and primary stent placement.

Fig. 7.6* is the baseline angiogram of a thrombus filled graft.

Angiogram of the excellent result following Possis Angiojet™ and stent placement of mid-graft lesion.

Figure 7.6 *continued*
*g) Result of RCA graft stenting. *,**) Aspiration thrombectomy with the Angiojet™.*

Case 6. Grafts

77-year-old woman. Hypertension; hypercholes-
terolaemia; family history. Inferior MI 1992.
CABG surgery 1992: vein grafts to LAD, OM and
RCA.
Recurrent, limiting angina.

Catheter findings: Moderate LV; patent grafts
but significant stenosis in native LAD beyond
anastomosis.

Procedure: Right Amplatz 2 guide (8F); 0.014"
high torque floppy wire. 3.0 mm monorail
balloon—1 inflation to 6 atm. No stent.

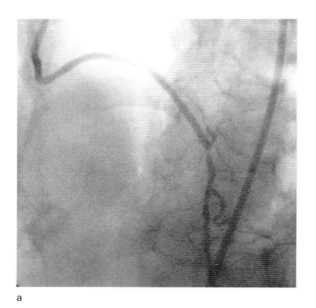 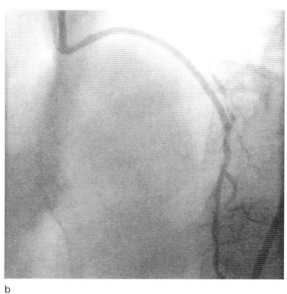

a   b

Figure 7.7
LAD graft angiogram. a) Post-anastomosis lesion. b) Final result post balloon dilatation.

Case 7. Grafts

52-year-old man. High cholesterol; ex-smoker. Inferior MI 1993. CABG surgery 1996: LIMA to LAD, vein grafts to RCA and OM. Required re-do grafting 4/97 with radial artery to LAD (LIMA occluded).
Further admission with unstable angina.

Catheter findings: Good LV; occluded RCA (dominant); severe proximal disease in LAD; occluded proximal circumflex; VGs to circumflex and RCA patent with good run-off. LIMA occluded.
Stenosis at insertion of radial artery graft into LAD.

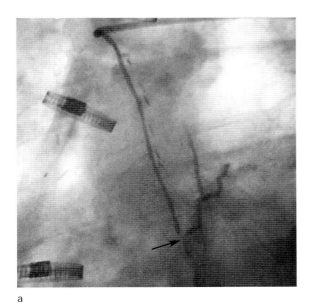

a

Figure 7.8
Radial artery graft to LAD. a) Anastamosis lesion.
b) Balloon positioning. c) Result.

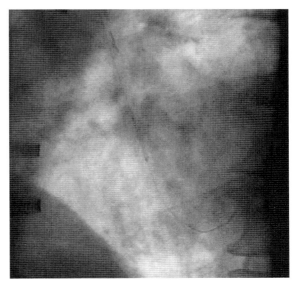

b

c

Christopher J White:

In these cases I would have selected either a Judkins right guide catheter or a left graftseeker with an extra-support guidewire to facilitate potential stent placement. Distal anastomosis lesions are frequently composed of fibrointimal hyperplasia, and statistically yield the best results, compared to other graft lesion locations, following angioplasty. My strategy would have been to perform 'provisional' stenting in these lesions, and I would have been happy to leave a 'stent-like' balloon result.

Editors' note

Several new devices and technologies are available to treat vein graft disease, particularly with a view to reducing rates of distal embolization and no reflow. The Percusurge system has already been mentioned and the Cordis AngioGuard™ is also now available. A third novel technology is the *stent graft™* by Jomed.

This is now described and illustrated by **Stephan Baldus** and **Christian W Hamm**.

Christian W Hamm and Stephan Baldus:

The coronary *stent graft* device represents a new and promising strategy for the treatment of lesions in aortocoronary venous bypass grafts. These *stent grafts* are stents covered by a poly-tetrafluorethylene (PTFE) membrane fixed between two layers of stent struts (Fig. 7.8d).

The membrane bears the potential for effectively holding thrombotic debris on the vessel wall and thereby reducing distal embolization. Preliminary data suggest a reduction in the incidence of in-stent restenosis. For stent implantation we would recommend using low pre-dilatation pressures to prevent mobilization of thrombus material. The stent itself should be deployed using high inflation pressures (> 10 atm) to overcome the reduced compliance of this device.

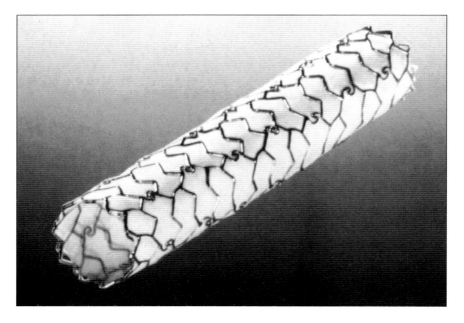

Figure 7.8d
Jomed stent graft™.

Case 8. Grafts

73-year-old man. Hypercholesterolaemia, hypertension, smoker, coronary artery bypass grafting 1984, presenting with angina pectoris class III. Coronary angiogram revealed de novo lesions in both the vein grafts to the LAD and to the RCA.

Procedure: The patient underwent a one stage procedure treating focal lesions in bypass grafts anastomosed to the RCA and LAD. While the lesion in the LAD graft was treated by two conventional stents, the lesion in the RCA graft was treated by a stent graft.
LAD graft: 7F guide; standard 0.014″ guidewire, pre-dilatation with a 3.5 mm balloon (7 atm) (VIVA, Boston Scientific). Two AVE Microstents (Medtronic™) were implanted (3.5 mm × 12 mm),

stent implantation pressure 10 atm. A satisfactory post-procedural result is seen (Fig. 7.9c).
RCA graft: 7F guide; 0.014″ Hi Torque Sport guiding wire; pre-dilatation with a 3.5 mm balloon (9 atm). Implantation of a 9 mm stent graft (3.5 mm) (Fig. 7.9d), stent implantation pressure 16 atm. Acceptable post-procedural result (Fig. 7.9e).

Follow-up: After 6 months the patient underwent re-angiography which revealed severe in-stent restenosis in the lesion treated by the conventional stents (Fig. 7.9f) whereas the lesion covered by the stent graft showed only minimal lumen loss (Fig. 7.9g).
QCA revealed 81% versus 8% in-stent restenosis in the lesion treated by the conventional stents versus the stent graft lesion.

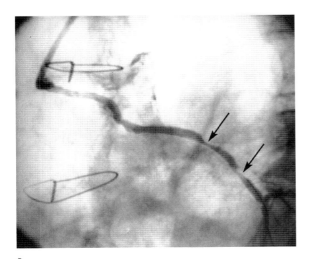

a

Figure 7.9a–f
a) LAD vein graft with distal lesions. b) RCA graft mid-course lesion.

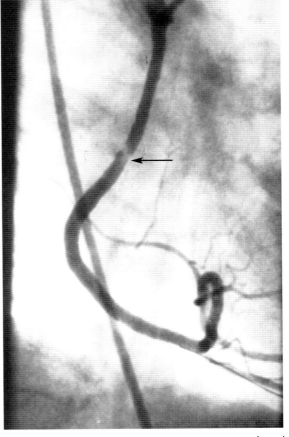

b

continued

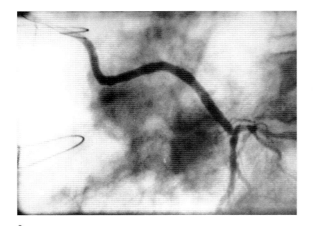

c

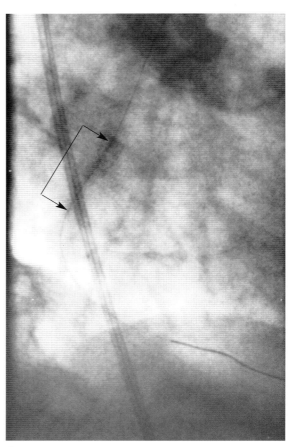

d

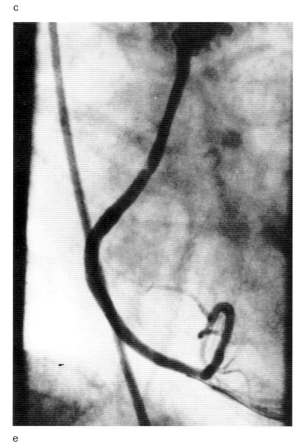

e

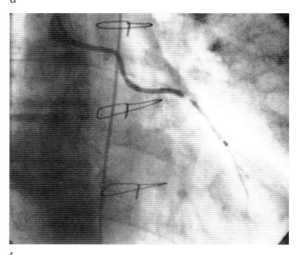

f

Figure 7.9 *continued*
c) Result after stenting with 2 standard stents in LAD graft. d) Positioning of stent graft in RCA graft.
e) Result at 6 month follow-up. f) 6 month follow-up angiogram showing severe stenosis in LAD graft.

Case 9. Grafts

43-year-old man. Acute chest pain, known coronary artery disease. Diabetes, hypercholesterolaemia, smoker, prior MIs 1991 and 1997, emergency PTCA 1999 in cardiogenic shock.

Catheter findings, 1999: LAD and RCA occluded, proximal Cx 95% stenosis. PTCA and stent Cx with stabilization of haemodynamic function. Following the procedure he remained asymptomatic and coronary bypass surgery was discounted, owing to an apparent lack of graftable distal vessels.

Catheter findings, 2000: In-stent occlusion Cx with TIMI 0 distal flow (Fig. 7.10a). LVEDP 50 mmHg, BP 110/60 mmHg and PAP 50/25 mmHg, heart rate of 120 b.p.m.

Procedure: Emergency IABP and PTCA Cx; 3.5 mm × 20 mm Omnipass balloon, and 4.0 mm AngioGuard™ distal embolization protection device placed (Figs 7.10b,c and appearance of device open Fig. 7.9d). After PTCA Cx, flow at AngioGuard™ poor. 0.014″ guidewire passed to maintain access, AngioGuard™ removed. Immediate flow of TIMI 3 (Fig. 7.10e) associated with reduction in symptoms. Angiogram after intracoronary nitrates (Fig. 7.10f). Patient made uneventful immediate recovery. As distal RCA and LAD patent, CABG undertaken 1 week later.

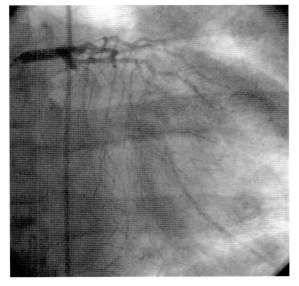

a

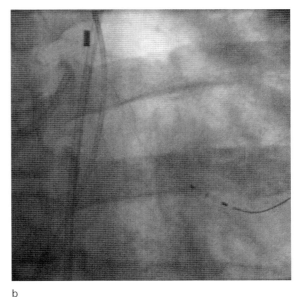

b

Figure 7.10a–f
LCA angiogram. a) In-stent occlusion Cx with TIMI 0 distal flow. b,c) Omnipass balloon and AngioGuard™ device placed.

continued

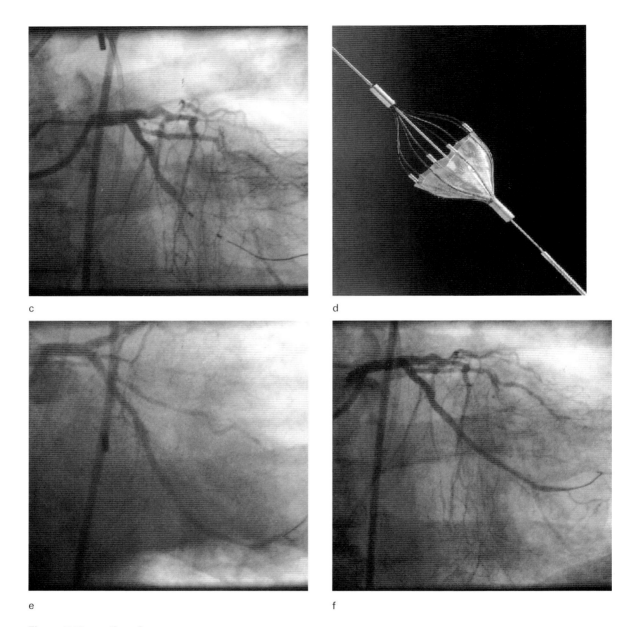

c

d

e

f

Figure 7.10 *continued*
d) Device opened. e) Immediate flow of TIMI 3. f) Following intracoronary nitrates.

Christopher SR Baker and Martin T Rothman comment on the AngioGuard™:

Prevention of distal embolization in a critical lesion is an attractive concept. Using a distal protection device that needs to be advanced across the potentially friable territory is worrisome, however. This case demonstrates that this technology can be used in such a case and that the distal 'umbrella' catches material that would otherwise embolize and perhaps cause vascular obstruction and possibly lead to cardiac enzyme elevation reflective of myocardial damage. In a situation of single remaining vessel disease this protection is relatively more important.

The current first-generation distal protection devices are bulky, somewhat rigid and require care in their use. None the less they demonstrate proof of the principle that they can and do capture potential emboli, thus probably reducing the extent of the myocardial injury.

Clinical trials are awaited that demonstrate the clinical value of this new generation of interventional devices.

Reference

1. Sirnes PA, Golf S, Myreng Y, et al. Stenting in chronic coronary occlusion (SICCO): a randomised, controlled trial of adding stent implantation after successful angioplasty. J Am Coll Cardiol 1996;28:1444–1451.

8
Direct stenting

Stent insertion without pre-dilatation carries the appeal of quicker cases that cost less in terms of finance and radiation exposure. There is the theoretical possibility that there is less trauma to the vessel wall and the suspicion that, particularly in vein graft disease, there will be less distal embolization. Such appealing concepts have led to great interest in this technique. Randomized and controlled trials are currently underway but the current body of evidence is based upon observational data. Certain clinical features and types of lesion are thought to be favourable for direct stenting, including:

- Recent history of angina and especially acute coronary syndromes
- Vein grafts
- Lack of calcification

Most interventionists by now have had the sinking feeling when the stent will not access or cross the lesion and becomes loose on its delivery system, and at these times, if we are honest, we ask 'why am I trying to do this?' The response to such a crisis is an important component to the skill of the direct stent enthusiast because clearly it can make the difference as to whether the stent is lost or not. There are certainly a variety of disadvantages to direct stenting:

- Difficulty with visualization and positioning once the stent delivery system encroaches into the lesion
- Failure to pre-dilate can lead to deployment of a stent that is suboptimal in diameter or length
- Stent expansion is sometimes incomplete at the heart of a tough lesion, thus necessitating the use of a non-compliant balloon (negating the cost advantage)

It seems likely that direct stenting has a niche in the armamentarium of the interventionist and forthcoming trials may help to pinpoint the nature of that niche. As can be seen from the response of our experts to these illustrative cases, there is not yet consensus!

In this chapter we sought the expert opinion of **Bernard Chevalier, Thierry Lefevre** and **Martin T Rothman.**

Bernard Chevalier provides this background to the direct stenting argument

Indications and contraindications

The major indication for direct stent implantation is, above all, a validated indication for systematic stenting, particularly in BENESTENT-like lesions. By contrast, I consider there to be three categories of contraindication.

Those related to the risk of the lesion being undilatable:

- Age > 75 years
- Stable angina related to a target lesion of more than 6 months' duration

Those related to the lack of systematic stenting indication:

- Small vessel (< 2.6 mm)

Those related to the complexity of stenting procedure:

- Chronic occlusion
- Bifurcation lesion
- Highly calcified artery and/or lesion.

Thus, in my opinion, by this classification the optimal use of direct stenting does not exceed 50% of all PTCA procedures.

Potential benefits

Some are obvious:

- Less use of disposable products
- Shorter procedure time
- Less radiation exposure

Some remain to be validated:

- Less longitudinal wall injury
- Lower stent/lesion ratio
- Lower late reintervention rate, particularly for diffuse in-stent restenosis

Randomized studies are in progress to confirm our preliminary mid-term results.

Potential risks

The major additional risk related to this technique is the placement of a stent in an undilatable lesion. However, I am convinced that good clinical and angiographic selection may avoid this problem. In 1000 patients treated with this technique in my centre, there have been only three cases of incomplete deployment, with a final residual stenosis between 30 and 40% (as assessed by off-line QCA analysis). The final pressure after direct stenting is absolutely the same as for the conventional pre-dilatation technique, with 1% of stents deployed at a pressure exceeding 16 atm. Post-dilatation is limited to 20% and, particularly if high pressure is necessary, is performed with a shorter balloon to avoid the 'dog-bone' effect at the two ends of the balloon.

Specific complications

Taking into account these different key points, we have been able to limit the major adverse cardiac event rate during in-hospital stay at 1.2% in simple and moderately complex lesions. Moreover, the rate of minor adverse events such as stent loss (0.3%), balloon rupture (0.2%), and incomplete deployment (0.3%) are extremely low and certainly compete with the results of the conventional stenting technique. These results also reflect the lower complexity of the lesions addressed by the direct stenting technique.

Tips and tricks

- Good clinical and angiographic selection of patients and lesions (particularly the flow must allow a good assessment of the lesion)
- Good back-up from the guiding catheter
- Choice of a low profile, well secured stent on a flexible delivery device with good clearance in the guiding catheter
- Selection of a stent that is not oversized and long enough to have at least 2 mm of safety margin at both ends of the stenosis
- Use of landmarks to facilitate stent placement, particularly if it is thought that there will be no contrast flow through the stenosis when the stent is across
- Progressive inflation to nominal pressure, and then we would recommend waiting for at least 45 to 60 seconds before deciding to go above this, because the simultaneous processes of dilatation and deployment require time!
- In case of persistent indentation, go slowly to higher pressure but not over the rated burst pressure (RBP) of the delivery device. In case of continuing resistance at RBP, we would remove the delivery device and post-dilate with a balloon of the same length as the stent.
- In case of failure to cross, *do not push a lot*: remove the stent and pre-dilate

The vein graft issue

The precise question of direct stent implantation in saphenous vein graft lesions is interesting. In fact, we may anticipate both a specific benefit (entrapment of thrombus or soft atheroma material with stent struts) and also a specific risk (higher rate of a fibrous lesion, particularly in ostial and proximal graft lesions, with a consequent higher risk of resistance to dilatation). There must therefore be very careful selection before direct stenting is used to treat a vein graft lesion. Moreover, the crossing of the stent must be easy and in case of resistance, the stent should be removed in order to avoid force, which increases the risk of distal embolization.

Case 1. Direct stenting

70-year-old woman. High cholesterol; family history. Limiting angina with inferior ST depression on ETT.

Catheter findings: JR4 8F guide; 0.014″ high torque floppy wire; AVE GFX 3.5 mm × 12 mm stent directly (Figure 8.1b).

Bernard Chevalier:

This case is interesting because it is not a typical case to begin with the direct stenting technique. We have here four factors that are associated, in my practice, with direct stenting failure: age > 70, stable angina, pre-PTCA MLD < 0.5 mm, and use of the AVE GFX stent. However, this direct stent implantation is quite successful and this example demonstrates the difficulty in predicting direct stenting success. Extension of direct stenting to this kind of indication must be restricted to high volume operators with a large experience of direct stenting in easier circumstances.

Thierry Lefevre:

New-generation hand-crimped stents have made direct stenting possible. Frequent users of this technique (> 30% of cases) have reported encouraging preliminary results, claiming that in case of impossibility to cross the lesion it is always possible to pull the stents back into the guiding catheter without any complication. Furthermore, direct stenting may be associated with shorter procedural duration and possibly fewer dissections and a lower restenosis rate.

We think that gaining 5 minutes is not very important in a patient in whom a stent is implanted for life. Consequently, in patients with stenosis of native arteries and stable angina, considering the risk of incomplete deployment of the stent or stent loss, this technique will remain experimental until we are able to demonstrate that it may reduce the risk of complication and restenosis.

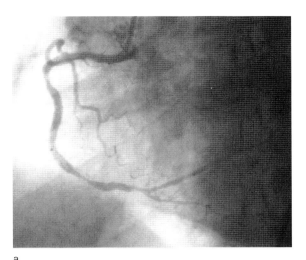

a

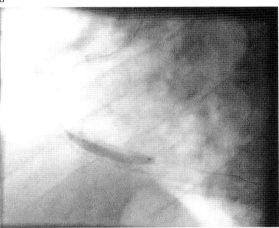

b

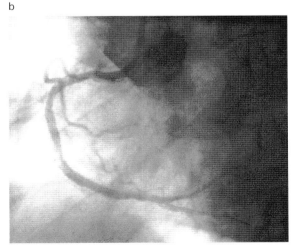

c

Figure 8.1
RCA angiogram. a) Lesion in distal horizontal portion of vessel. b) Balloon and stent inflation. c) Result.

Case 2. **Direct stenting**

79-year-old man. Hypertension. Acute inferior MI complicated by complete heart block. Chest pain continued despite thrombolysis.

Catheter findings: Moderate LAD disease; unobstructed circumflex; dominant RCA with tight distal stenosis.

Procedure: JR4 (8F); 0.014″ high torque floppy wire. Direct stent to lesion with 3.5 mm × 15 mm Cordis CrossFlex™ to 12 atm (Figure 8.2b). Some clot seen in distal vessel (Figure 8.2a). Abciximab (ReoPro®) given.

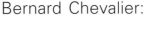

Bernard Chevalier:

A typical case for direct stent implantation: an acute myocardial infarction lesion with a high probability of little resistance to stent access, with TIMI III flow despite a severe stenosis. Our experience of direct stent implantation in acute myocardial infarction is very positive, with a lower rate of no-flow after stenting compared to conventional stenting.

However, as in this example, the rate of distal embolization is not decreased. Direct stenting in acute MI is associated with a higher rate of TIMI III flow at the end of the PTCA and is my favourite strategy in this situation *if baseline flow*

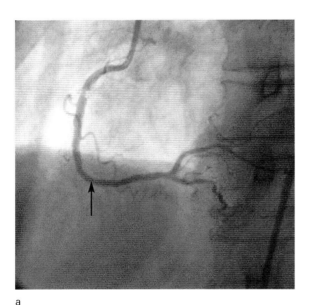

a

Figure 8.2
RCA angiogram. a) Proximal discrete lesion and distal probable clot at arrow. b) Proximal balloon and stent inflation. c) Result, small residual waist in proximal stented segment but clot has cleared from the RCA and embolized to posterior LV branch.

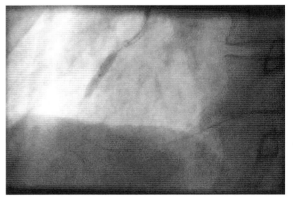

b

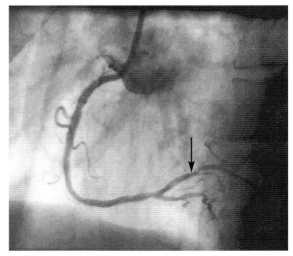

c

or flow after wire crossing is good enough to allow a satisfactory evaluation of the lesion length. Age is a limitation of direct stenting and here we can see a slightly incomplete relief of the indentation at the site of the lesion.

Thierry Lefevre:

The problem is different in unstable syndromes and in saphenous vein grafts, because in the presence of thrombus or very soft or friable plaque, the risk of slow flow, no reflow and/or distal embolization is high.

In cases of unstable angina or acute MI, when we suspect the presence of thrombus direct stenting is our preferred approach because it probably decreases the risk of distal emboliza-tion and slow flow or no reflow.

Stent selection is crucial. With coils stents and, less frequently, with multicellular stents, we have observed some prolapse through the stent (thrombus or very soft plaques). For this reason we have been using tubular stents that allow good plaque coverage (NIR™, beStent™, Crown).

In case of failure, it is very important, before pulling the stent back into the guiding catheter, to obtain a good alignment between the stent and the guiding catheter. We frequently perform inflations at 0.3 atm to 0.5 atm to avoid contact of the stent with the guiding catheter edges.

Editors' note

If the stent/balloon combination needs to be removed because the device will not reach or cross the target lesion then we recommend that the guide catheter be pulled back from the coronary ostium before the stent/balloon is removed from the coronary in those cases where guide catheter engagement is not perfect for stent recovery. Our practice is to displace the guide catheter until it is virtually vertical in the ascending aorta. This will prevent the guide catheter being 'pulled' into the coronary ostium as the stent is pulled back out of the vessel and it will therefore prevent the stent being stripped off the balloon and deposited in the ostium. This manoeuvre will also allow the stent/balloon to orientate itself so that it is co-axial with the guide catheter lumen and will ease the passage back into the guide catheter.

Several more cases are provided by Thierry Lefevre for discussion

Case 3. Direct stenting

65-year-old man. Hypertension, high cholesterol. Acute inferior MI. Onset to admission: 11 hours.

Catheter findings: Ejection fraction 42%, inferior akinesia, occlusion of the mid-RCA with thrombus.

Procedure: JR6 F guide; 0.014" ACS BMW wire; Hand-crimped NIR™ 9 cells 3.5 mm × 32 mm without pre-dilatation mid-RCA 14 atm and hand-crimped NIR™ 9 cells 3.5 mm × 0.25 mm without pre-dilatation distal RCA 12 atm.

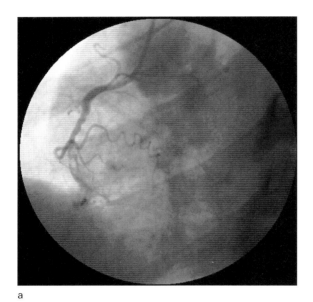

a

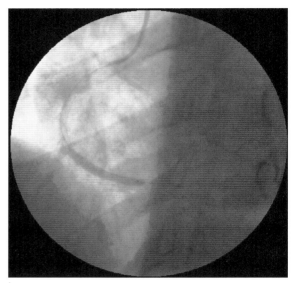

b

Figure 8.3
RCA angiogram. a) Occluded mid-RCA with sluggish distal flow. b) Balloon and stent inflation. c) Result.

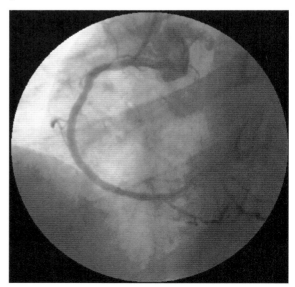

c

Thierry Lefevre:

This case demonstrates that direct stenting can be practised in long segment disease as well as the BENESTENT type lesion. The operator's choice to undertake this type of approach in this case is governed by the fact that there is a short clinical history and the angiographic appearance is in the main that of clot in the vessel rather than long-segment atheromatous disease.

Whilst there is a residual stenosis proximal to the proximal stent this is not flow limiting and was left. Usually in these cases distal flow, and the calibre of the distal vessel, improve in appearance and can be much improved even within 24 hours. Dilatations downstream should be resisted unless there is important limitation in flow, as these features are often due to residual clot that will usually resolve in the presence of flow.

Case 4. Direct stenting

43-year-old man. Smoking, high cholesterol. Acute anterior MI, cardiogenic shock. Onset to admission: 4 hours.

Catheter findings: Occlusion of the distal left main (Figure 8.4a).

Procedure: IABP and ReoPro®. JL4 6F guide; left main thrombus and TIMI II flow to the LAD and CX; 2 ACS BMW wires one to LAD and a second to protect the circumflex. Hand-crimped beStent™ 3.5 mm × 25 mm (left main and proximal LAD) 12 atm; proximal left main optimized with a 4.0 mm Tacker balloon 14 atm.

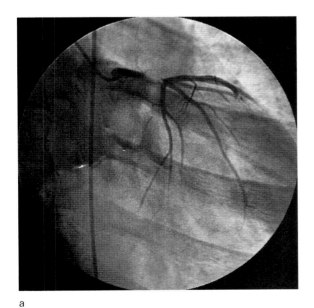

a

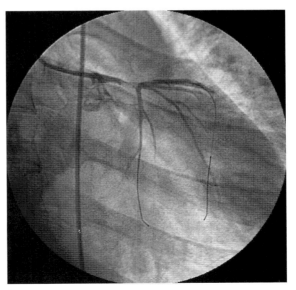

b

Figure 8.4a–f
LCA angiogram. a) Distal LM occlusion. b) Clot delineation improved with passage of guidewire to LAD.

continued

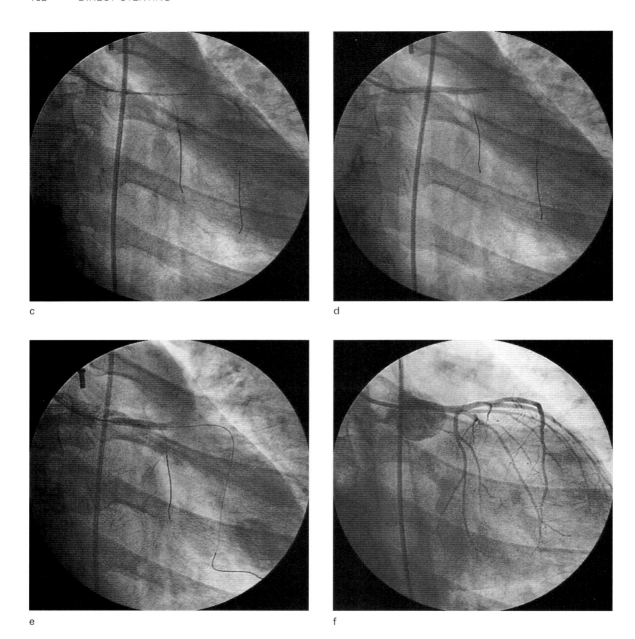

c

d

e

f

Figure 8.4 *continued*
c) Two guidewires, one in LAD and one in CX. Stent advanced to LM and proximal LAD. d) Balloon and stent inflation to LM and LAD, CX wire trapped outside stent. e) Post-dilatation. f) Final result with wires removed.

Martin T Rothman comments on Thierry Lefevre's case:

An excellent example of the use of direct stenting, partly because it demonstrates the value of the technique when 'time is of the essence'. The procedure can be very fast and can be critical when flow needs to be re-established urgently and with a level of assurance not guaranteed by balloon angioplasty alone.

The use of two guidewires here is more than simply cosmetic, it is good sense, given the appearance of the clot which seems to be straddling the circumflex artery origin. Given this appearance it seems quite likely that clot may embolize down the circumflex, or worse still be 'snowploughed' into the origin of the circumflex, thereby closing the vessel and possibly rendering the origin difficult to locate in an emergency.

The procedure is undertaken completely in the LM and LAD, as the circumflex was unaffected.

Case 5. Direct stenting

47-year-old man. High cholesterol. Family history of coronary disease. Acute anterior MI, cardiogenic shock. Onset to admission: 4.5 hours.

Catheter findings: Occlusion of the proximal LAD, with visible thrombus. Thrombotic lesion of the first marginal with TIMI III flow.

Procedure: IABP and ReoPro®. EBU4 6F guide catheter; ACS BMW wire allowing correct assessment of lesion length; direct stenting with hand-crimped NIR™ 3.5 mm × 25 mm. Despite Reopro®, lesion of the marginal remained unchanged at 12 hours. Direct stenting with DUET 3.0 mm × 23 mm.

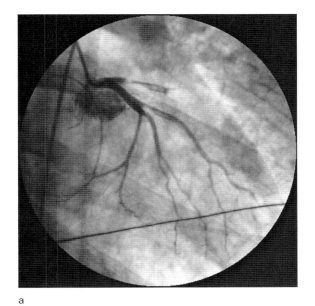
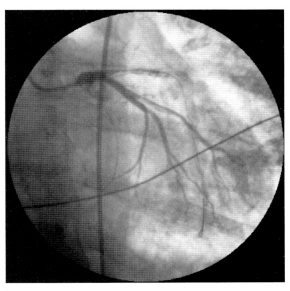

a   b

Figure 8.5a–g
LCA angiogram. a) Occluded LAD proximally. b) Guidewire to LAD flow seen into LAD.

continued

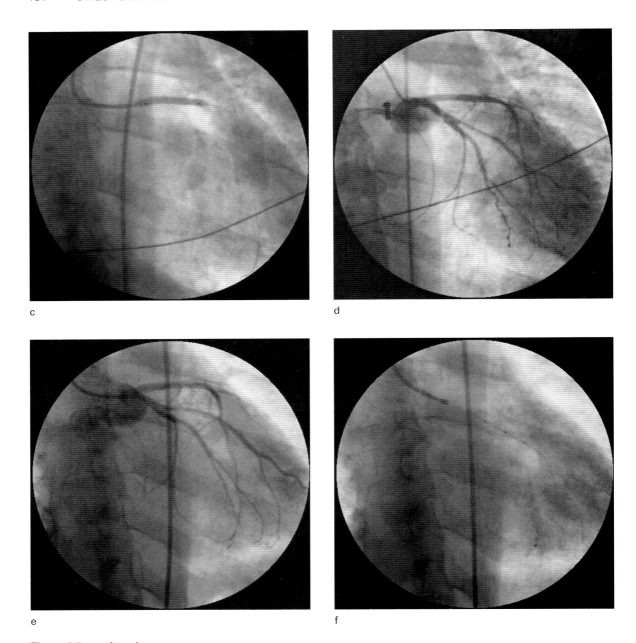

Figure 8.5 *continued*
c) Balloon and stent deployment. d) End result in LAD. e) Lesion in OM. f) Balloon and stent positioning in OM.

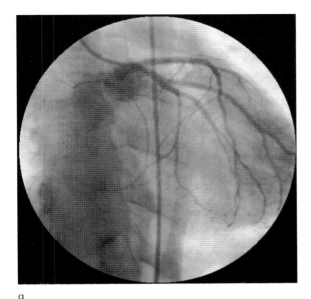

g

Figure 8.5 *continued*
g) Final result.

Martin T Rothman comments on Thierry Lefevre's case:

Run-off into the mid-LAD can be seen and the culprit lesion length can be estimated to be reasonably short. The clinical history is also short and thus this may be a good case for direct stenting. It is also worth appreciating the guide catheter position and making an assessment of possibility of removing the balloon stent delivery system if the stent will not cross. This guide catheter appears to be well aligned with the LM and looks reasonable both for providing support and for allowing for system removal, if necessary.

It may be a reasonable decision to leave the OM vessel on the first occasion, as it is not usually considered important from the LV impairment point of view. However, when a patient without prior symptoms develops cardiogenic shock it may sometimes be necessary to undertake quite extensive revascularization at the first intervention to ensure as much perfusion to the ischaemic myocardium as possible. The risk of extensive treatment is much reduced by stent implantation and as the patient is going to have abciximab anyway we consider it reasonable to do all the major lesions at one sitting. The need for extensive intervention may be necessitated because of failure of the haemodynamic state to improve.

Case 6. Direct stenting

67-year-old man. Smoker, high cholesterol. CABG in 1990: saphenous vein graft to the right coronary artery, saphenous vein graft to the marginal and LIMA to the LAD. Acute inferior MI, Killip Class 1.

Catheter findings: Thrombotic occlusion of the saphenous vein graft.

Procedure: Multipurpose 8F guide, 0.014″ ACS Balance Heavy weight. Acolysis 6 minutes; direct stenting of the lesion with a hand-crimped NIR™ 4.0 mm × 25 mm.

Martin T Rothman comments on Thierry Lefevre's case:

In saphenous vein grafts, direct stenting is also the preferential approach, although it is not always possible, especially in old saphenous vein grafts. Here we see the appearance of a recent occlusion in the vein graft with clot in the distal end of the column of contrast. This is an encouraging sign as it may signal an easy passage across the stenosis, but it does not indicate the length of the clotted segment beyond. It must also be remembered that the distal end of the column of contrast does not necessarily coincide with the site of the lesion. It may well be the case that the site of stenosis is very distal to the interface position we see, and the vein graft is loaded with clot. Thus the passage of the wire may be easy through the proximal segment and then may hang up distally. If the guidewire hangs up distally then it may be worth using an over-the-wire balloon and taking it down to the end of the straight section of the wire in the graft and using the balloon as a platform from which to hunt for the lumen. If there is doubt about the location of the tip of the wire it is worthwhile removing the guidewire and injecting dilute contrast down the wire lumen to highlight the distal anatomy.

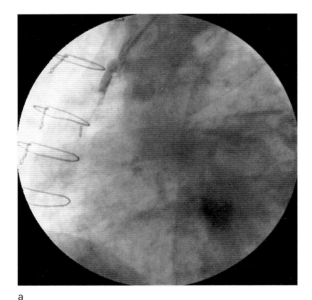

a

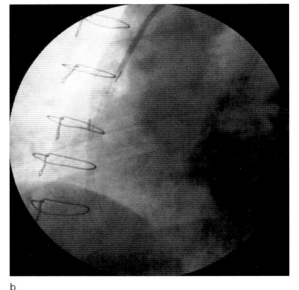

b

Figure 8.6a–e
RCA graft angiogram. a) Proximal occlusion with 'clot' appearance. b) Acolysis catheter in proximal graft: the device is activated and low frequency ultrasound emitted from the catheter tip with the theoretical advantage of clot lysis.

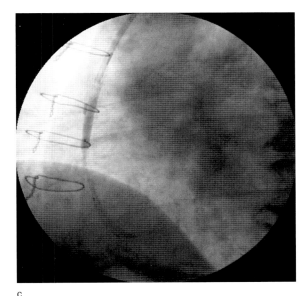

c

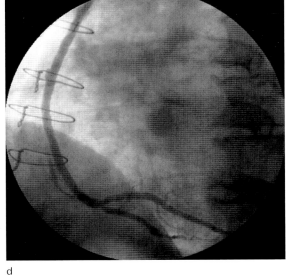

d

Figure 8.6 *continued*
c) Contrast column now longer. d) Post direct stenting.
e) Good distal vessels without evidence of embolization.

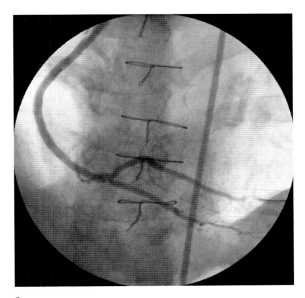

e

With the information gained, one may more confidently cross to the distal vessel.

In this case it would appear that the stenotic lesion was fairly close to the distal end of the column of contrast, so direct stenting was acceptable. This can often be confirmed to be the situation immediately after passing the guidewire, as this allows enough contrast to flow distally to allow definition of the downstream anatomy.

As was indicated by Bernard Chevalier in his opening remarks, there are good theoretical reasons for direct stenting in vein grafts, clot entrapment by the stent being one of them, to encourage this approach. Also there is a theoretical argument that says that the fewer passages across the clot-laden area the less likely it is that embolization will occur. I am not impressed by these arguments, as it seems unlikely that thin steel filaments are going to trap much clot, and it seems likely that much of the clot will be extruded between the stent struts at the time of stent deployment and will embolize immediately or soon after, irrespective of whether it was a direct stenting case or balloon followed by stent. My argument for direct stenting in this situation is that it is very convenient, achieves a good result, and is often quick—a point of value if many lesions are to be undertaken at the same intervention.

All of the above not withstanding, this is an excellent result in a potentially very difficult situation.

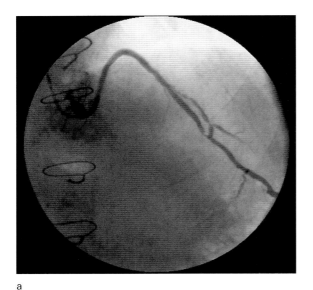

a

Case 7. Direct stenting

69-year-old man. Smoker, high cholesterol level. CABG in 1987: saphenous vein graft to the LAD, saphenous vein graft to the right coronary artery. Dilatation and stenting of the proximal and mid-part of the saphenous vein graft to the LAD for unstable angina. New episode of unstable angina 6 months later.

Catheter findings: No restenosis but a new lesion at the distal anastomosis.

Procedure: LCB 6F guide. 0.014″ ACS BMW. Direct stenting with hand-crimped beStent™ 3.5 mm × 15 mm.

Martin T Rothman comments on Thierry Lefevre's case:

There is a good example of direct stenting of the region of a graft immediately proximal to the anastomosis site of the vein graft to the LAD. The distal end of the stent has been placed into the native LAD distally and, as one might expect, the retrograde flow to the proximal LAD is unimpaired. The only point at issue here is guide catheter support, and if this catheter does not provide support then an Amplatz right may sometimes give the support required.

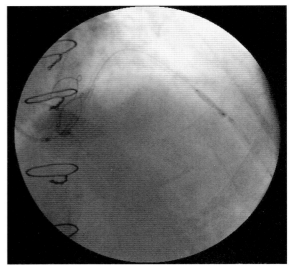

b

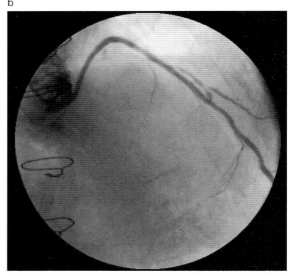

c

Figure 8.7
LAD graft angiogram. a) Lesion seen just proximal to graft insertion into LAD. b) Balloon and stent deployment. c) Result.

Also, guidewire positioning is important. It is necessary to have the 'strong' portion of the guidewire in the lesion to facilitate crossing of the stent. It is usually a mistake not to have the guidewire as distal as it will go, ensuring the strongest available portion of the guidewire is across the lesion, facilitating crossing.

9
Ostial disease

Ostial lesions often deprive the operator of one of the sound platforms for angioplasty success; good guide catheter support. Delivery of devices is therefore fraught with technical difficulty. The positioning of an ostial stent whilst pushing on the guidewire and withdrawing the guide catheter slightly is one of intervention's most subtle manoeuvres. The potential for difficulty in these cases encourages idiosyncrasies in technique to as great an extent as any other lesion type!

Comment on these ostial disease cases is provided by **Christian W Hamm, Stephan Baldus** and **Martin T Rothman**.

Case 1. Ostial disease

70-year-old woman. NIDDM; family history; hypercholesterolaemia. Limiting exertional angina.

Catheter findings: LV moderate; Left coronary unobstructed; RCA as shown.

Procedure: Multipurpose (8F) guide; standard 0.014″ wire; extensive pre-dilatation with 3.0-mm monorail balloon. Then three stents deployed, overlapping from distal vessel: (a) ACS MULTI-LINK® 3.5 mm × 25 mm; (b) NIR™ 3.5 mm × 32 mm; (c) ACS MULTI-LINK® 4.0 mm × 25 mm. The proximal ACS MULTI-LINK® was positioned so that it extended right back to the ostium by disengaging the guide catheter.

Martin T Rothman:

This case demonstrates the difficulty of guide catheter support when treating an ostial or very proximal lesion. Good guide catheter engagement can sometimes be problematic, as the tip of the catheter can impinge on the lesion and occlude flow or damage the plaque. If there is serious risk of damage to the ostial lesion then over-enthusiastic searching for good engagement can be dangerous. In these situations it is worth orientating the guide catheter towards the ostium of the vessel and then hunting for the lumen with the wire, my preference to start being the high torque floppy (Guidant). This wire has excellent tip control and will not usually damage the plaque. Even in difficult engagements, as in this example, it is possible to 'stabilize' the guide catheter using the guidewire. Once the wire is through the lesion it can be manipulated to the distal vessel without much guide catheter support. The guide catheter can then be orientated to the vessel as the balloon is advanced across the lesion. Once across, and with the balloon inflated, a contrast injection can help define local landmarks for the subsequent stent deployment.

For ostial lesions it is important to cover the ostium, and to do this successfully it is necessary to have the stent a little way out into the aorta. Care needs to be taken to understand the anatomy of the patient, as the anatomy varies significantly. It is worth while taking time to locate the optimum angiographic view, and it is sometimes sensible to inflate the balloon with

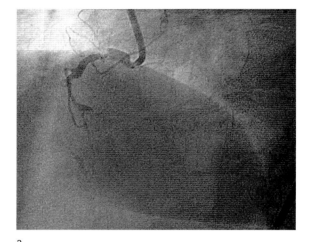

a

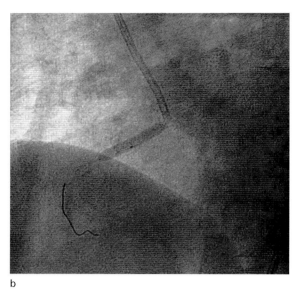

b

Figure 9.1
RCA angiogram. a) Guide catheter not well engaged, pointing a bit inferiorly. Proximal, mid and distal disease seen. b) Balloon inflated with guide catheter displaced away from ostium. c) Final result.

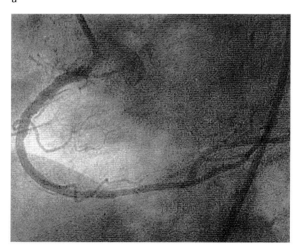

c

the proximal end some way out into the aorta, with the guide catheter backed away from the ostium, and use the waist or inflection point in the balloon to learn the true position of the aorto-ostial junction. Next the position of the proximal end of the stent with reference to the marker bands on the balloon should be examined. It is valuable to know whether the proximal end of the stent is immediately adjacent to the proximal marker band, or whether there is a gap. With this information it is easier to 'visualize' the position of the stent in the aorto-ostial junction. Finally it is useful to

use a stent with good radio-opacity so that its location can be seen directly, rather than inferred from the position of the balloon marker band.

With the stent positioned in the aorto-ostial junction, test injections should be undertaken to confirm position. In my experience it is more common to have the stent too far in, than too far out. The stent should be inflated gradually so that the position of the waist caused by the lesion can be viewed, to confirm the accuracy of the placement. Also, a contrast injection should be recorded, as this can confirm the stent location. It may indicate the need for a second stent more proximally if the stent has been placed too distally. Once the stent has been deployed it is worth taking the balloon back so that it is half in the stent, and then inflating again to high pressure to flare the proximal end of the stent. Care should be taken when pulling the balloon back during this manoeuvre as there is a tendency for the guide catheter to be pulled into the ostium and this can damage the proximal end of the stent before it is flared. Once the stent has been flared the guide catheter will usually sit nicely into the ostium. However, if it will not locate easily then it is likely that the tip is tripping over the proximal part of the stent in the aorta. In this case either use the balloon, placed into the stent, to help locate the guide catheter or abandon the use of the guide catheter and use a diagnostic catheter to confirm the final appearance.

On very rare occasions it proves impossible to engage the guide catheter, and it is also impossible to 'throw' the guidewire from the disengaged guide catheter into the vessel. In these situations, having tried numerous guide catheters, one can consider a different approach: say from the brachial or radial artery. As a technique of last resort it has sometimes proven possible to use a diagnostic catheter from which to pass the guidewire into the vessel. Then the diagnostic catheter can be removed, leaving the guidewire in the vessel, and a guide catheter can be passed to the ostium over this guidewire; it is not as difficult a manoeuvre as it sounds!

Case 2. Ostial disease

72-year-old man. Ex-smoker; hypertension. 1983 single vein graft to LAD. Severely limiting angina.

Catheter findings: Good LV; unobstructed dominant RCA; occluded proximal LAD; large circumflex with stenosis in OM1; patent vein graft to LAD with significant ostial disease.

Procedure: Multipurpose (8F) guide; 0.014″ high torque floppy wire. Direct stent to ostium and proximal portion of graft using Guidant Duet ACS MULTI-LINK® 4.0 mm × 23 mm stent. Further inflation within stent using a 4.5 mm Chubby™ balloon.

Martin T Rothman:

Similar considerations to those described in the previous case pertain here. In this case bony landmarks can be used for reference as to the ostial position of the graft. Likewise the bend in the balloon at the ostium at the time of the pre-dilatation, if this were undertaken, would help with defining the aorto-ostial location. The position of the guide catheter defines the aorto-ostial position in this case, and direct stenting is therefore an option. However, bear in mind the fact that aorto-ostial junctions can be quite difficult to dilate as they do not always release easily, so this may be a situation where under-deployment of the direct stent may be expected, and where post-dilatation may be

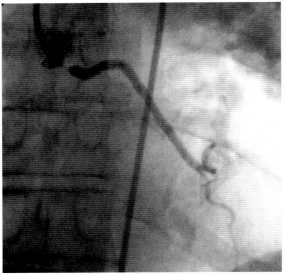

a

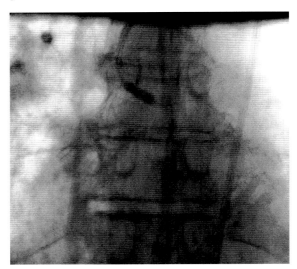

b

Figure 9.2
LAD graft angiogram. a) Ostial disease. b) Balloon and stent deployment. c) Post-dilatation of ostial portion of stent.

c

required. This was indeed the case here, and the Chubby™ balloon was used both to optimize the result and to flare the proximal end of the stent. Again, be aware that the optimization balloons can have high profile after use and can thus pull the guide catheter into the proximal end of the stent if care is not taken. In this situation it is worth backing the guide catheter away from the ostium by some distance before attempting to remove the Chubby™ balloon from the stent, so as to avoid the guide catheter 'diving' into the stent.

Case 3. Ostial disease

65-year-old man. Hypercholesterolaemia, hypertension, current smoker, presenting with angina pectoris CCS class III. Coronary artery bypass grafting 1985 with venous bypass grafts to the LAD, first diagonal, circumflex artery and first marginal branch.

Catheter findings: Single subtotal lesion in the venous bypass graft to the LAD.

Procedure: Guiding catheter LCB 7F, guiding wire Extra Support 0.014", pre-dilatation 3.5 mm Rocket balloon (AVE), inflation time 55 seconds,

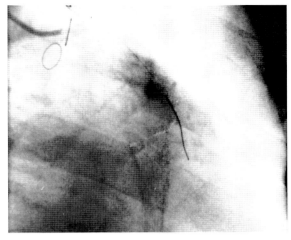

c

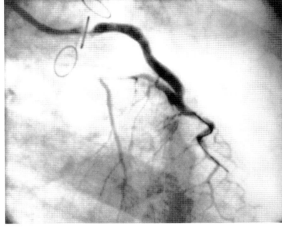

a

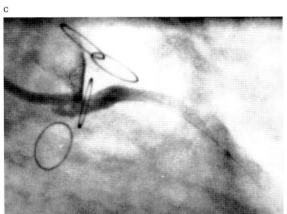

d

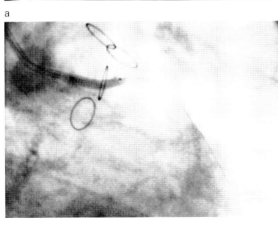

b

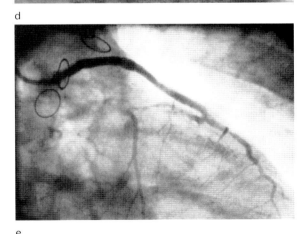

e

Figure 9.3
LAD angiogram. a) Aorto-ostial lesion. Note markers were in aorta wall, and limit of contrast in sinus of graft. b) Balloon inflation. c) Stent graft in ostium of LAD. d) Early result. e) 6 months angiogram showing good medium-term patency.

inflation pressure 4 atm; stent implantation Jostent Coronary Stent Graft® 3.5 mm × 12 mm; total inflation time 55 seconds, 18 atm. The post-procedural angiographic result was acceptable.

Christian W Hamm and Stephan Baldus:

Ostial lesions represent a challenging lesion subgroup in native vessels as well as bypass graft lesions, since elastic recoil often leads to a late luminal loss and restenosis even after stent implantation.

This case illustrates stent implantation of a Jomed stent graft described previously in the section on vein graft management (see page 78). It is characterized by a PTFE membrane sandwiched between two aligned layers of stainless steel. Elastic recoil and in-stent restenosis appears to be effectively reduced by the membrane.

In this case the location of the ostium is conveniently marked by a radio-opaque suture placed by the surgeon at the time of the original operation. The balloon inflation is undertaken half in and half out of the graft. The stent graft can be visualized on the angiogram (Fig. 9.3c) and the result in Fig. 9.3d shows an excellent immediate result. The 6 months' follow-up (Fig. 9.3e) angiogram in this asymptomatic patient shows a maintained patency somewhat unusual for an ostial lesion and suggests a benefit from using the Jomed stent graft.

Case 4. Ostial disease

66-year-old man, presenting with angina pectoris class III, cardiac risk factors; hypercholesterol-aemia, hypertension, ex-smoker, renal insufficiency.
The patient had undergone coronary artery bypass grafting in 1989 and 1994.

Catheter findings: Patent LIMA to the LAD but occluded vein grafts anastomozed to the RCA and the circumflex. The native RCA showed severe ostial disease.

Procedure: Guiding catheter: JR4, 9F guiding wire c-soft 0.014″; Rotablator burr size initially 1.5 mm, followed by 2.25 mm.
PTCA after Rotablator using Extra Support guidewire 0.014″; balloon: 4.0 mm × 20 mm Presario™ (Medtronic); maximum inflation 18 atm; total inflation time 180 seconds.
Stent implantation using Jomed Coronary Stent Graft™, length 9 mm mounted on a 4.5 mm Presario™ balloon, maximum inflation pressure 19 atm, total inflation time 42 seconds. Optimization after stent implantation to overcome incomplete expansion of the stent centre using 4.5 mm × 10 mm Viva (Boston Scientific), maximum inflation pressure 20 atm; total inflation time: 60 seconds.

Christian W Hamm and Stephan Baldus:

This patient had an ostial lesion seen in Fig. 9.4a, and underwent successful Rotablation (Fig. 9.4b) and PTCA but had recoil immediately (Fig. 9.4c) and finally received a PTFE membrane covered Jomed stent graft seen after implant (Fig. 9.4d) to give an excellent immediate result (Fig. 9.4e).

The elective follow-up angiogram after 6 months revealed a favourable long-term angiographic result (Fig. 9.4f), again a somewhat unusually good result suggesting a benefit from use of the Jomed stent graft.

Figure 9.4
RCA angiograms. a) Ostial RCA disease.
b) Rotablation of ostial lesion. c) Recoil of ostial lesion.
d) Stent graft being positioned in ostium of RCA.
e) Good immediate result. f) Six month angiogram.

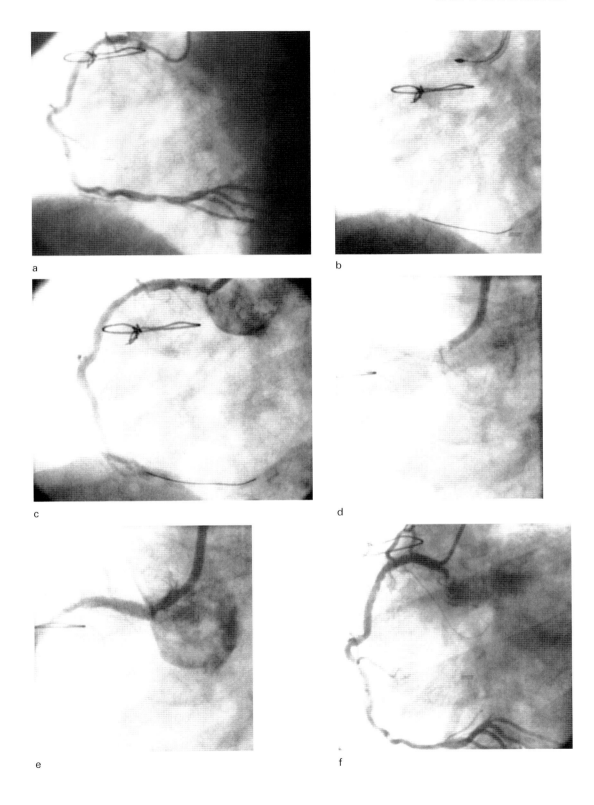

10
Acute coronary syndromes

Acute coronary syndromes represent an increasing proportion of the workload of the interventionist. For patients who present with unstable angina and non-Q wave MI, PTCA and stenting offers a rapid and efficient means of terminating ischaemia and facilitating the patient's discharge on less medication. In some places that have more favourable logistics than the average centre in the UK, particularly the United States, patients presenting with acute myocardial infarction are frequently treated by primary angioplasty rather than thrombolysis. The recent data suggest that such patients benefit from stenting rather than balloon alone. Furthermore, the desire to limit myocardial damage around the time of acute MI has led, entirely appropriately, to a rapid increase in the number of patients referred for revascularization who have not responded to thrombolysis or who have clearly reinfarcted following apparently successful chemical recanalization of the infarct-related vessel.

The immediacy and spectacular symptomatic effects of such cases are a potent drive to their increasing numbers. Such considerations are increasingly being coupled to evidence that suggests prognostic benefit. It is thus inevitable that we will continue to deal with ever-increasing numbers of such patients. This workload appears to be associated with higher complication rates than for elective cases, although the original complication rates that are quoted are undoubtedly out of date with the introduction of stents, improved anti-platelet therapies, including abciximab, and increasing operator experience. Each case is different, but acute coronary syndromes throw up some testing questions for the interventionists, some of which are listed below and can be illustrated by the cases we have selected.

- Should ReoPro® be routine in all these cases?
- Is there concern about the use of ReoPro® soon after thrombolysis?
- Should we wait if there is a large thrombus load?
- Should the 'culprit' vessel be tackled only in the acute setting even if there is treatable disease elsewhere?
- Is stenting obligatory in such cases?
- Would it be better to pre-dilate only when necessary?
- What is the best strategy for 'no reflow'?
- Are some stents better than others in the presence of thrombus?
- Is there a place for devices that offer mechanical dissipation, removal or distal entrapment of thrombus?

Expert comment on acute coronary syndrome management is provided by **Michael Kutryk** and **Harvey White**.

Case 1. Acute coronary syndromes

48-year-old man. Smoker; family history. January 1997 acute inferior MI treated with streptokinase. Further episode of pain with ST elevation inferiorly eleven days later.

Catheter findings: LV: mild inferior wall hypokinesis only; unobstructed LCA; RCA as shown.

Procedure: JR4 guide (8F); 0.014" high torque floppy wire; 3.0-mm monorail balloon. AVE GFX 3.5 mm × 18 mm to 12 atm.

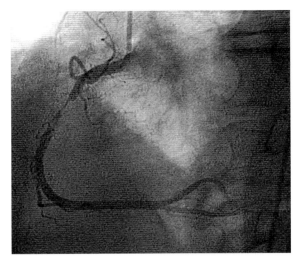

a

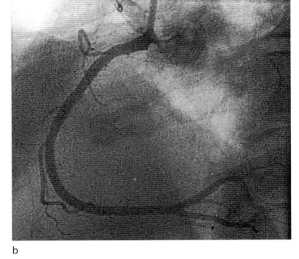

b

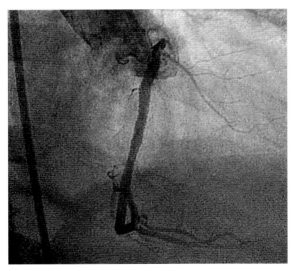

c

Figure 10.1
RCA angiogram. a) Proximal RCA disease. b) Post-stent angiogram in LAD projection. c) Post-stent angiogram in RAD angiogram.

Michael Kutryk:

Prior to treatment, this is a complex, relatively tight lesion. The JR4 catheter appears to be well engaged and probably provides adequate support for this relatively straight segment. However with newer-generation low-profile tightly crimped stents, direct stenting might be considered and an extra-support guide catheter might be preferable. In this case, the lesion was pre-treated with a 3.0 mm balloon, which is rather generous. If the intention were to proceed to stenting, pre-dilatation with a smaller balloon would minimize the risk of dissection.

The choice of stent is reasonable. The second generation GFX stent has a reasonably high hoop strength (> 15 psi in independent testing) although tubular stents such as the MULTI-LINK® or R Stent™ have higher radial force (hoop strength of R Stent > 25 psi) and are less likely to recoil. Tubular stents would give a better appearing final result with less plaque prolapse. In the final image, there appears to be a small waist in the stented segment. High pressure post-dilatation with a low-compliance, short balloon should be performed to improve the apposition of the stent to the vessel wall and improve the final appearance. This is also important as the stent appears to be under-sized. The distal segment appears to be larger than 3.5 mm (compared to the 8F, 2.7 mm guiding catheter). This lesion could easily have accommodated a 4.0-mm diameter stent. The length of the stent used in this case appears appropriate.

There should be a low threshold for the use of abciximab in this situation. This is a complex lesion with a large thrombus and/or plaque burden.

Harvey White:

I would prefer to use a 6F guide, and I would not pre-dilate with good guide support, little calcium and reasonable landmarks for positioning of the stent. The length of the stent is appropriate, but it may be slightly under-sized. I would not use ReoPro® in this case.

Case 2. Acute coronary syndromes

43-year-old man. Ex-smoker; family history; high cholesterol; diabetes mellitus.
Acute anterior MI (treated with streptokinase) followed by post infarct angina.

Catheter findings: Discrete tight stenosis in LAD; remaining coronaries unobstructed; moderate overall LV function.

Procedure: JL4 8F, 0.014″ high torque floppy wire. 3.5-mm monorail balloon; 3.5 mm × 16 mm NIR™.

Michael Kutryk:

The lesion in this case is a relatively short B1 lesion. The JL4 catheter appears to fit well, and probably provides adequate back-up for this segment. If the intention was to proceed to stenting, then the 3.5 mm balloon for pre-dilatation is over-sized and will only increase the risk of serious dissection. For pre-dilatation it is necessary only to create a channel large enough for the stent to pass, so it would be prudent to select a smaller balloon. The pre-dilatation balloon length should be equal to or less than that of the predicted stent length. As there are no major side branches associated with this lesion, the choice of a NIR™ stent is reasonable. The length and diameter of the stent appears appropriate.

As this patient is diabetic, treatment with abciximab is supported by the 6-month (decreased target vessel revascularization rate) and 1-year (reduced death rate) findings of the EPISTENT trial.[1,2]

Harvey White:

I would choose a different guide catheter (XB/Voda) for better guide support, and again I would not pre-dilate. A short NIR™ stent of the appropriate size has been used and a good result obtained. ReoPro® would be appropriate in this case, given the presence of diabetes and post-infarction angina.

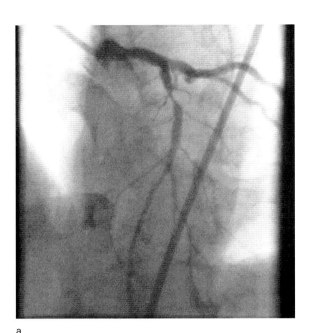

a

b

Figure 10.2
LCA angiogram. a) Tight proximal LAD lesion. b) Result after stenting.

Case 3. Acute coronary syndromes

28-year-old man. Hypertension; hypercholesterol-aemia; family history. Pain and ST elevation in inferior leads treated with streptokinase (peak CK 2800 IU). Continued to have pain and transferred to angiography laboratory with ST elevation in inferior leads.

Catheter findings: Good overall LV with inferior hypokinesis; mild LAD disease; occluded OM from dominant circumflex; non-dominant unobstructed RCA.

Procedure: Abciximab (ReoPro®) bolus and infusion. JL4 8F guide; 0.014″ high torque floppy wire with 3.0 mm monorail balloon inflated once to 8 atm. No stent.

Michael Kutryk:

In this case of rescue angioplasty good back-up support is essential in order to optimize the chances for success. For this reason, an Amplatz guide catheter may have been a better first choice. In the setting of a total occlusion, a high torque floppy guidewire is a good selection. Another wire that seems to give consistently good results in these types of lesions is the Choice PT™. The 6-month results of the Zwolle Myocardial Infarction Trial[3] and the PAMI Stent Randomized Trial[4] indicate that primary stenting offers significant advantages over PTCA, especially by decreasing the need for subsequent infarct-related artery revascularization procedures. The results of the Controlled Abciximab and Device investigation to Lower Late Angioplasty Complications (CADILLAC) trial will hopefully confirm these results. Thus, primary stenting may be preferable in the setting of an acute MI. It is difficult, however to judge the length of the lesion from these two images. If the diseased segment is long (> 20 mm), stent implantation may result in prohibitively high 6-month restenosis rates.

Since the prothrombotic effects of thrombolytic agents have been mainly attributed to platelet activation, the use of abciximab is generally considered to be a valuable approach in

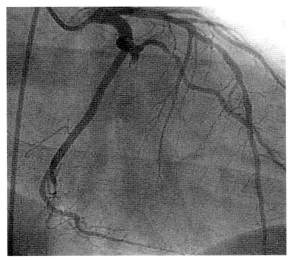

a

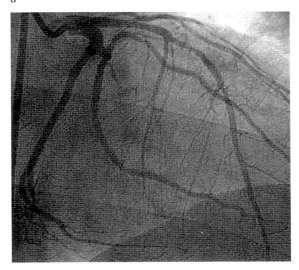

b

Figure 10.3
LCA angiogram. a) Occluded proximal OM. b) Result after balloon only.

rescue angioplasty. There are some data to support this. The EPIC AMI subpopulation, which included 22 patients who had rescue PTCA after failed thrombolysis, found that the 6 month composite endpoint (death, AMI and TVR) was significantly reduced with the use of abciximab. The combination of fibrinolytic therapy and GP IIb/IIIa inhibition to 'facilitate' percutaneous coronary interventions is specifically being examined in TIMI-14, SPEED, and GUSTO IV, and early results appear promising. The optimum dose of both thrombolytic and anti-platelet agents has yet to be determined.

The risk for no-reflow is high in this situation and the operator should be prepared for the intracoronary administration of nitrates, verapamil or adenosine. There are no data to suggest that the relative youth of this patient should be a factor in the decision of whether or not to stent.

Harvey White:

An XB/Voda guide catheter would be better than a JL4. I would stent all reasonably sized occluded arteries and, unless it was a bail-out situation, I would not give ReoPro® so soon after strepto-kinase. Streptokinase reduces fibrinogen levels, and blockade of the binding of platelet IIb/IIIa receptors to fibrinogen with ReoPro® may increase the risk of major bleeding. The age of the patient would not affect my decision to stent.

Case 4. Acute coronary syndromes

74-year-old man. Hypercholesterolaemia. Acute pain with anterior T-wave changes. 7 days later further acute pain with ST elevation anteriorly, treated with streptokinase; he was transferred for angiogram.

Catheter findings: Poor overall LV function; occluded LAD; significant circumflex lesion; unobstructed (dominant) RCA.

Procedure: JL4 8F guide; 0.014" high torque floppy wire with 3.0 mm over-the-wire balloon for disobliteration and then multiple inflations to a series of stenoses. Thrombus seen in vessel. No stent. Abciximab (ReoPro®) infusion.

Michael Kutryk:

Similar to the preceding case, this is an example of rescue PTCA. A guide catheter with better back-up support should be considered. As in the previous example, given the results of the reported trials, a case can be made for primary stent implantation. However, the fact that multiple inflations were required to a series of stenoses suggests an excessively long lesion that may make stent implantation a less attractive option. The presence of intracoronary clot should not affect the decision to stent, particularly in the era of GP IIb/IIIa inhibitors. In light of the considerable clot burden, consideration should be given to treatment with a thrombectomy device such as the X-SIZER or the AngioJet™. Although the results of the PAMI-2 trial indicated no major clinical benefit for routine IABP insertion during primary PTCA in high-risk patients, one still might consider prophylactic insertion of a balloon pump in this elderly gentleman with poor LV function and two-vessel disease.

The use of abciximab in the setting of rescue percutaneous interventions is currently under investigation. However, early data suggest an added beneficial effect as outlined in the previous example.

It is generally accepted that only the culprit lesion be treated in the setting of an acute infarction. Treatment of the circumflex lesion at the same setting only increases the risk of complications. The circumflex lesion should be treated at a later date if clinically indicated. For the future treatment of the circumflex lesion, abciximab can still be used with judicious monitoring for allergic

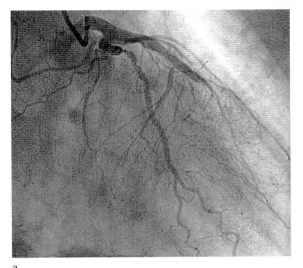

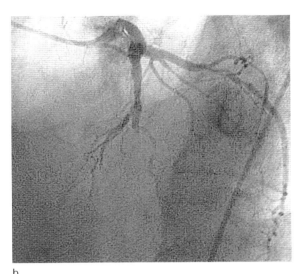

a

b

Figure 10.4
*LCA angiogram. a) Occlusion of mid-LAD seen in
RAO projection. b) Occlusion of mid-LAD seen in LAO
projection. c) Result.*

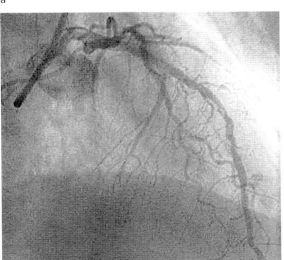

c

reactions, attenuated efficacy, and immune-
mediated thrombocytopenia.

Harvey White:

This patient has extensive disease and would be
a good case for the use of ReoPro®, but I would
be cautious in that the patient has just received
streptokinase. I would use an XB/Voda guide
catheter and electively stent. There is a significant residual stenosis after ballooning with
thrombus. Given the poor overall LV function, a
poor result in the LAD, the contrast load, and the
length of the circumflex stenosis, I would probably defer treatment of the circumflex stenosis
to a second procedure.

Case 5. Acute coronary syndromes

53-year-old woman. Family history; ex-smoker; hypertension.
Non-Q wave infarction with recurrent chest pain and inferior territory ECG changes.

Catheter findings: Good LV function; unobstructed left coronary artery; dominant RCA occluded distally.

Procedure: JR4 8F; 0.014″ high torque floppy wire backed up by 1.5 mm over-the-wire balloon. Further dilatation with 2.5-mm monorail balloon followed by Cordis CrossFlex™ 3.0 mm × 15 mm stent.

Michael Kutryk:

The JR4 guide seems to engage well and provides adequate back-up support for this right coronary artery. The type of stent chosen is adequate for this lesion. The decreased distal run-off of this vessel makes appropriate diameter sizing of the stent difficult. The operators in this instance chose a stent with an appropriate, perhaps generous, diameter. The stent seems to be well placed, and traverses the narrowest part of the lesion. The spot stenting literature supports this approach as being optimal treatment for this type of lesion. Distal to the stented segment, the PDA rapidly tapers, and distal treatment would probably not add any incremental benefit while increasing the risk of dissection.

The use of adjunctive abciximab should be considered.

Harvey White:

The diseased anatomy involved here is an inferior surface branch which, from the still frames, looks like a 2.5 mm rather than a 3.0 mm vessel, and I'm unsure of the length of the stenosis. It looks shorter than the length stented. I would not electively stent this small vessel. A balloon plus ReoPro® would be a reasonable approach.

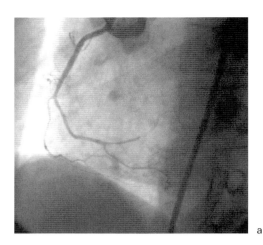

a

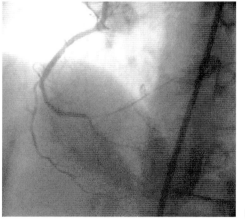

b

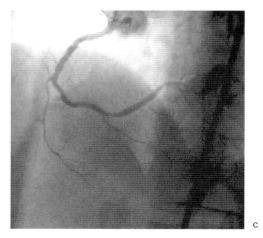

c

Figure 10.5
RCA angiogram. a) Distal occlusion in the PDA vessel. b) Following balloon dilatation. c) Following stent implantation.

Case 6. Acute coronary syndromes

60-year-old man. NIDDM; ex-smoker; hyper-cholesterolaemia; family history.
Acute anterior MI 3 weeks before transfer. He was treated with streptokinase and he then redeveloped pain with ST elevation anteriorly, and was given tPA. He was then mobilized but continued with post-infarct angina.

Catheter findings: Moderate overall LV function with anterior hypokinesis; RCA unobstructed; moderate circumflex lesion; LAD as shown.

Procedure: Voda 3.5 left 8F; 0.014″ high torque floppy wire; 3.0 mm monorail balloon; 3.5 mm × 25 mm ACS MULTI-LINK® stent to 10 atm.

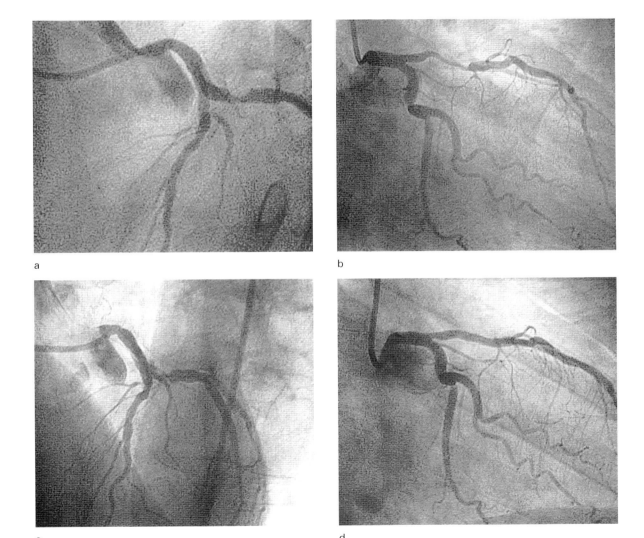

a

b

c

d

Figure 10.6
LCA angiogram. a) Proximal LAD lesion seen in LAO cranial projection. b) Lesion seen in RAO causal projection. c) Result following stent implantation, LAO projection. d) Result following stent implantation, RAO projection.

Michael Kutryk:

The operator's decision to use a guide catheter with extra back-up was good. Problems may be encountered with direct stenting in a lesion of this length, therefore pre-dilatation is indicated. A balloon smaller than 3.0 mm should have been chosen for pre-dilatation, in order to minimize the risk for dissection. As the stent was deployed at 10 atm, it might be wise to ensure optimal apposition of the stent to the vessel wall using IVUS or by higher pressure post-dilatation within the stent with a short, low compliance balloon. The MULTI-LINK® stent is a good choice as it possesses high radial strength, good side-branch access and optimum metal to artery coverage.

These favourable features are likely to have contributed to the preservation of the first septal branch after stent deployment. The choice of stent diameter is good, and the final result is excellent.

As this patient is diabetic, the use of abciximab should be strongly considered.

Harvey White:

This is an appropriate choice of guide catheter and stent, with a good result. Stenting without pre-dilatation would be appropriate. The circumflex stenosis should also be treated.

Case 7. Acute coronary syndromes

60-year-old woman. Ex-smoker; NIDDM. Recurrent ST elevation inferiorly 2 days after streptokinase for acute inferior MI.

Catheter findings: Unobstructed left coronary artery; RCA occluded.

Procedure: JR4 8F guide; 0.014″ high torque floppy wire and extensive dilatations with 3.0 mm monorail balloon. Overlapping stents from distal to proximal as follows:
(a) ACS MULTI-LINK® 3.5 mm × 35 mm to 10 atm; (b) ACS MULTI-LINK 3.5 mm × 35 mm to 12 atm.

'funnel' heralding the beginning of the total occlusion. If any difficulties were encountered, a Choice PT™ wire would be a good next choice. The choice of a 3.0 mm balloon for pre-dilatation is appropriate, given the final arterial diameter.

Abciximab is indicated in this situation, because of excessive stent length (70 mm) in a diabetic patient, particularly if intracoronary thrombus is apparent after pre-dilatation. It is in these types of lesion that spot stenting is being advocated in order to reduce the metal burden and possibly reduce the restenosis rate. The likelihood of restenosis with this amount of metal in a diabetic woman is extremely high, and unfortunately the operator will probably be faced with the difficult task of treating long, diffuse in-stent restenosis in subsequent months.

Michael Kutryk:

In this instance, the choice of guide catheter is appropriate. A high torque floppy wire is also a satisfactory choice, as there is an adequate

Harvey White:

In this case I would have considered using multiple short stents or, alternatively, I would have stented a slightly shorter length.

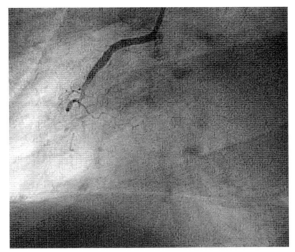

a

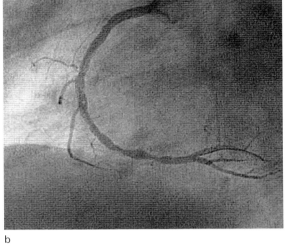

b

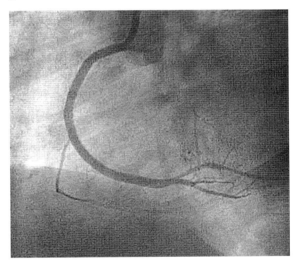

c

Figure 10.7
RCA angiogram. a) Occluded mid-RCA. Little centegrade flow to distal RCA. b) Clot appearance at site of orcalusum, and distal irregularity. c) Good final result.

Case 8. Acute coronary syndromes

49-year-old man. Smoker; family history. Abdominal surgery 3 weeks before presentation with chest pain and anterior ST elevation. Transferred from Accident and Emergency Department to catheter laboratory.

Catheter findings: Good LV with mild anterior hypokinesis; LAD occlusion; unobstructed coronaries elsewhere.

Procedure: JL3.5 8F guide; 0.014″ high torque intermediate wire backed up with 3.0 mm monorail balloon for disobliteration and then pre-dilatation. Cordis CrossFlex™ 3.0 mm × 15 mm just distal to first diagonal.

Michael Kutryk:

The choice of an intermediate weight, relatively stiff guidewire increases the risk of subintimal passage of the wire and the creation of a false lumen. A softer guidewire should be considered first. Although the CrossFlex™ stent is adequate for this lesion, a tubular stent may be a better choice. Stents such as the MULTI-LINK®, R stent™ or Jostent® provide higher hoop strength and less likelihood of plaque prolapse through the stent struts, yet maintain side-branch access.

The hazy appearance of the vessel distal to the stent in the final image suggests considerable thrombus burden. This is another case where the adjunctive use of abciximab should be strongly considered.

Harvey White:

I would have used a softer wire initially and a shorter stent, e.g. 9.0 mm or 12 mm.

Figure 10.8
LCA angiogram. a) Occluded LAD immediately after first diagonal. b) Appearance after passage of wire. c) Final result after stenting, with hazy appearance distal to stent.

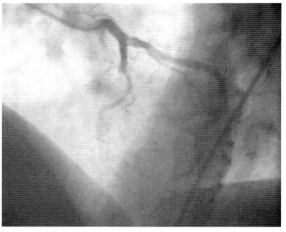
a

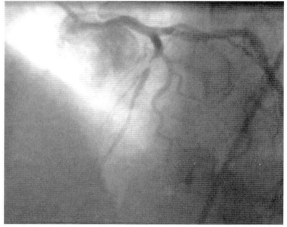
b

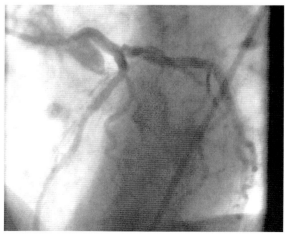
c

Case 9. Acute coronary syndromes

60-year-old man. Smoker; family history; high cholesterol. Inferior MI treated with streptokinase. Further pain with inferior ST elevation later that day.

Catheter findings: Good LV function with inferior hypokinesis; unobstructed LCA cross-filling the occluded dominant RCA.

Procedure: JR4 8F guide. 0.014" high torque floppy wire. Extensive dilatations with 3.0 mm monorail balloon. A lot of thrombus seen and no reflow achieved despite there being no obstructive lesions seen on angiogram. Abciximab (ReoPro®) overnight. Angiogram next morning showed good flow.

Michael Kutryk:

The ectatic nature of this right coronary artery and the high thrombus burden make this a good case for the use of a thrombectomy device such as the AngioJet™ or X-SIZER catheters, or distal embolism protection devices such as the PercuSurge Guardwire and Export Catheter. This vessel is not amenable to a stenting procedure. The risk for no-reflow in this situation is high, and the operator should be prepared to treat expeditiously if necessary with intracoronary nitrates followed by verapamil. If flow is not quickly re-established, high-velocity bolus injection of adenosine should be attempted.

In light of the large thrombus burden, the use of abciximab is justified in this situation.

The decision to re-look should be based purely on the clinical situation. There is no mention of the patient's post-angioplasty clinical condition, or whether the cardiac enzymes were elevated. If flow is promptly re-established, and the patient is stable clinically, then there is no need for a second look.

Harvey White:

This is a good case for ReoPro®, with an excellent result. Nitrates and verapamil should also be tried. Perhaps a larger balloon (3.5 mm) could also be tried to dissipate any thrombus present.

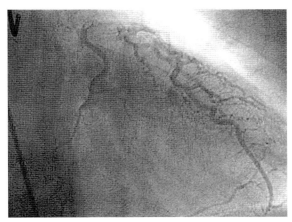

a

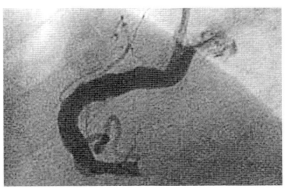

b

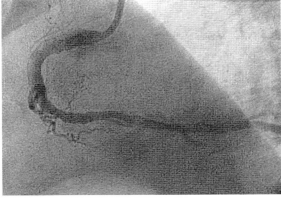

c

Figure 10.9
LCA angiogram. a) LCA injection showing collateral to RCA. b) RCA injection showing ectatic vessel with distal total occlusion. Not improved by balloon angioplasty. c) Angiogram 1 day later, after overnight ReoPro™.

Case 10. Acute coronary syndromes

67-year-old man. Ex-smoker; high cholesterol. Mitral valve replacement and vein graft to LAD 1991. Presented with unstable angina and anterior T wave inversion.

Catheter findings: Moderate LV function; proximally occluded LAD; non-dominant circumflex; diffuse disease in dominant RCA; recently occluded vein graft to LAD.

Procedure: Multipurpose guide 8F; 0.014″ high torque floppy wire. Multiple dilatations up and down graft with 3.0 mm monorail balloon. A lot of thrombus seen, therefore abciximab (ReoPro®) given. Stents deployed along diffusely diseased graft from distal to proximal:
(a) ACS MULTI-LINK® 3.5 mm × 35 mm; (b) ACS MULTI-LINK® 3.5 mm × 35 mm; (c) ACS MULTI-LINK® 3.5 mm × 35 mm; (d) ACS MULTI-LINK® 4.0 mm × 25 mm.

Michael Kutryk:

This very diseased vein graft would best be treated using a distal embolization protection device such as the PercuSurge Guardwire. Several centres advocate the routine use of the transluminal extractional atherectomy catheter (TEC) for the pretreatment of diffusely diseased saphenous vein grafts. The rationale for this combined approach is based on the idea that the TEC will partially remove plaque and thrombus, thereby reducing the potential for distal embolization. A substudy of the CADILLAC trial is assessing the validity of this approach, in the setting of adjunctive abciximab. The length of the stented segment puts this graft at high risk for restenosis.

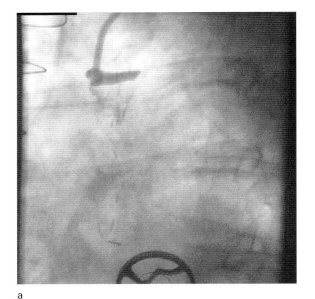
a

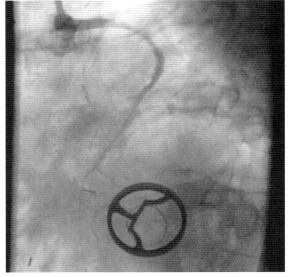
b

Figure 10.10a–e
LAD graft angiogram. a) Occluded graft, with cut-off appearance compatible with recent thrombotic occlusion. b) After passage of wire.

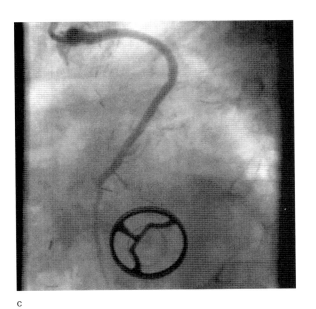

c

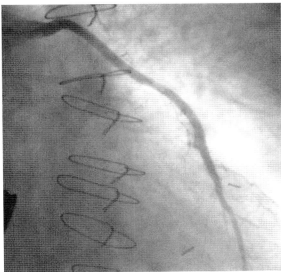

d

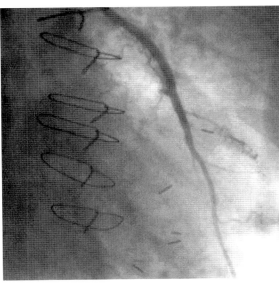

e

Figure 10.10 *continued*
c) After multiple stent insertions, LAO projection. d)
Result after stents, RAO projection. e) PA projection
to show anastamosis and distal graft appearance.

Harvey White:

This is a good case for the Angiojet™, and a sleeved stent (covered stent or stent graft) could also be tried. However, the graft is unlikely to remain patent in the long term, depending on how much focal atheromatous disease there is.

References

1. Marso SP, Lincoff AM, Ellis SG, et al. Optimizing the percutaneous interventional outcomes for patients with diabetes mellitus: results of the EPISTENT (Evaluation of platelet IIb/IIIa inhibitor for stenting trial) diabetic substudy. Circulation 1999;100:2477–2484.

2. Topol EJ, Mark DB, Lincoff AM, et al. Outcomes at 1 year and economic implications of platelet glycoprotein IIb/IIIa blockade in patients undergoing coronary stenting: results from a multicentre randomised trial. EPISTENT Investigators. Evaluation of Platelet IIb/IIIa Inhibitor for Stenting. Lancet 1999;354:2019–2024.

3. Suryapranata H, van't Hof AW, Hoorntje JC, de Boer MJ, Zijlstra F. Randomized comparison of coronary stenting with balloon angioplasty in selected patients with acute myocardial infarction. Circulation 1998;97:2502–2505.

4. Brener SJ, Barr LA, Burcehnal JEB, Katz S, Effron MB. Provisional stenting improves outcome of primary angioplasty independently of the use of abciximab. The RAPPORT trial. Circulation 1998;98:1–22.

11
Complications 1 – not dissections

A multitude of problems can arise during the performance of PCI and we have asked **Antonio Bartorelli** to comment on some non-dissection complication cases.

Case 1. Complications 1

72-year-old man. Ex-smoker. Long history of angina gradually becoming worse.

Catheter findings: Good LV; dominant RCA without significant stenoses; long segment of LAD disease.

Procedure: Amplatz left 2 guide; 0.014″ high torque floppy wire. 2.5 mm monorail balloon leading to local dissection followed by GFX 3.0 mm × 18 mm. Concern about step-down in size.

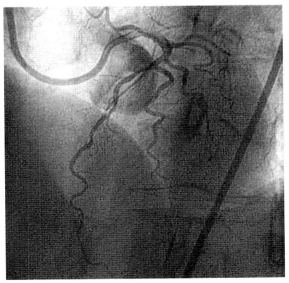

a

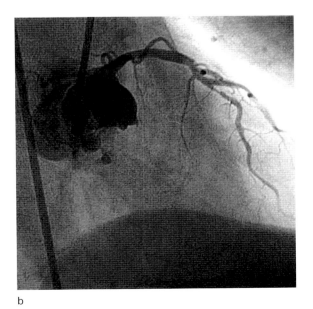

b

Figure 11.1a–d
LCA angiogram. a) LAD disease after 2nd diagonal, LAO projection. b) LAD disease after 2nd diagonal, RAO projection.

continued

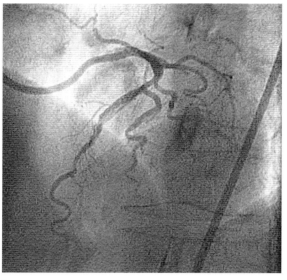 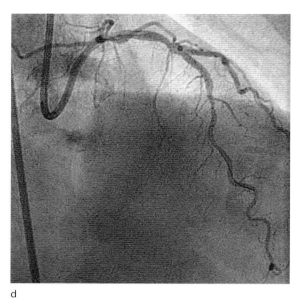

c   d

Figure 11.1 *continued*
c) Good result in lesion LAO. d) Good result, RAO. Step-down seen distal to stent.

Antonio Bartorelli:

This lesion involves the mid-portion of the left anterior descending coronary artery after the take-off of a large diagonal branch. As it often occurs in these cases, there is some tapering of the vessel lumen so that the diameter distal to the stenosis seems smaller than 3.0 mm. To avoid a step-down in size and the risk of dissection at the distal stent edge/vessel junction, I would have chosen a 2.5 mm delivery balloon and a stent with thinner struts than the AVE GFX. Post-dilatation of the proximal two-thirds of the stent with a short non-compliant 3.0 mm balloon would have assured good apposition against the vessel wall in the larger and more proximal portion of the vessel.

Case 2. Complications 1

52-year-old woman. Smoker; family history; hypertension. Deteriorating exertional angina.

Catheter findings: Good LV function; occlusion of circumflex; no other obstructive lesions.

Procedure: JL 3.5 guide 8F; 0.014″ high torque floppy wire backed up with 2.5 mm over-the-wire balloon, then Cordis CrossFlex™ 3.0 mm × 25 mm stent to 12 atm.

Antonio Bartorelli:

Significant vessel tapering often poses a problem when stenting long lesions. It is important to differentiate long lesions from diffuse disease. The latter is associated with increased risk of dissection at the distal edge of the stent, especially in case the delivery system is oversized and in vessel segments in which the angulation changes over 15° during the cardiac cycle (hinge or kinking points). When faced with lesion lengths of > 20 mm, significant tapering and a distal vessel of < 3.0 mm, my approach to reduce arterial wall injury is a stent delivery system sized 1 : 1 with the distal lumen dimension. High-pressure inflations with short balloons of larger size in the proximal mid-portion of the stented vessel or use of tapered balloons generally obtain stenting optimization without step-down and increased risk of dissection.[1]

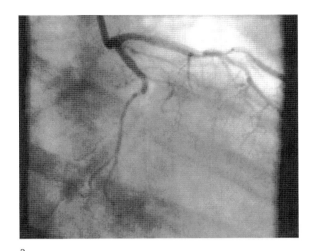

a

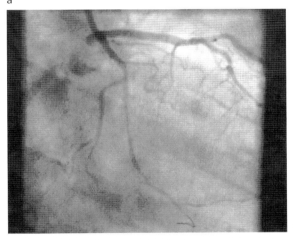

b

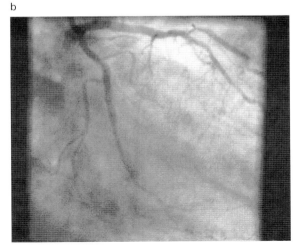

c

Figure 11.2
LCA injection. a) Occlusion of circumflex after small OM. b) After balloon dilatation vessel appears small. c) After stent deployment.

Case 3. Complications 1

59-year-old man. IDDM; family history. Exertional angina with inferolateral ST depression on ETT.

Catheter findings: Good LV; unobstructed circumflex and RCA; significant LAD disease.

Procedure: Left Voda 3.5 8F guide; 0.014″ high torque floppy wire; 3.0 mm monorail balloon. Following inflation to 8 atm, area of dilation looked hazy and was deemed too small to stent.

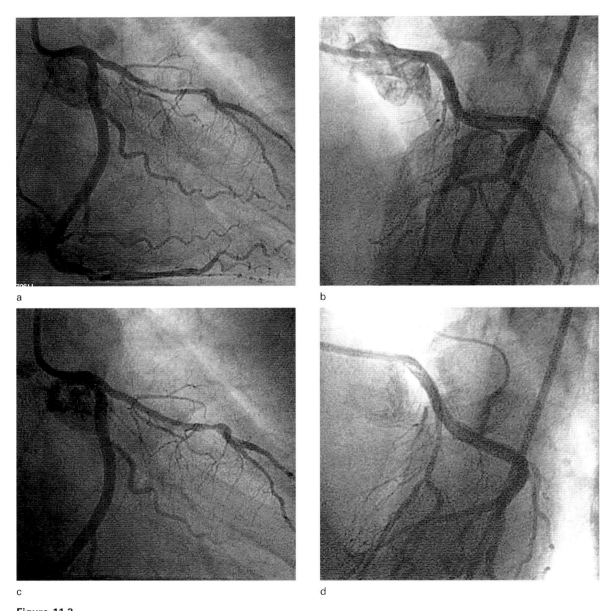

a

b

c

d

Figure 11.3
a) LAD disease seen in RAO projection. b) LAD disease seen in LAO projection. c) After balloon dilatation, RAO projection. d) After balloon dilatation, LAO projection.

Antonio Bartorelli:

Despite the small vessel size, stent implantation seems to be indicated in this case with a suboptimal PTCA result. Small vessel stenting has been associated with high angiographic and clinical success. In addition, the risk of stent subacute thrombosis has been shown to be low and comparable to that observed in > 3.0 mm vessels when an appropriate high-pressure deployment technique is used. Finally, the relative impact of stents on restenosis is actually better in a vessel of < 3.0 mm than in a vessel of > 3.0 mm. Use of new stents with dedicated design for small vessels and anti-thrombotic coatings such as the ByodivYsio™ SV or CarboSTENT™ 2.5 would have been my choice in this case. The presence of radio-opaque markers at stent edges in the latter device may allow more precise and safer intra-stent post-dilatation, especially in small vessels.

Case 4. Complications 1

71-year-old woman. Ex-smoker; high cholesterol. Severe limiting angina. One admission with unstable angina and anterolateral ST segment depression.

Catheter findings: Good LV function; dominant, unobstructed RCA; large diagonal vessel containing tight stenosis; rest of LCA unobstructed.

Procedure: JL4 8F; 0.014″ high torque floppy wire. Lesion pre-dilated with 2.5 mm × 10 mm

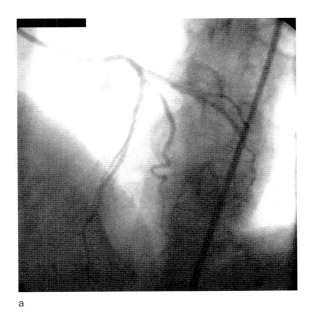
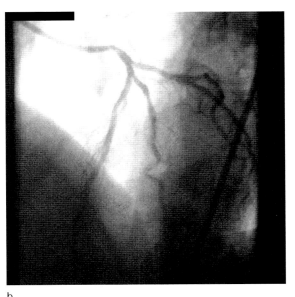

a   b

Figure 11.4a–g
LCA angiogram. a) Tight proximal diagonal stenosis. b) Result after stent deployment, new distal stenosis.

continued

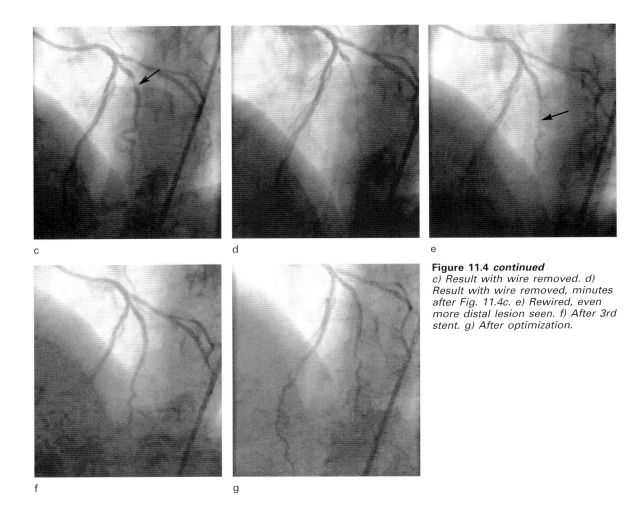

c

d

e

f

g

Figure 11.4 *continued*
c) Result with wire removed. d) Result with wire removed, minutes after Fig. 11.4c. e) Rewired, even more distal lesion seen. f) After 3rd stent. g) After optimization.

monorail balloon and stented with a 3.0 mm × 10 mm Cordis CrossFlex™. Excellent result until the wire was removed, when a tight narrowing was seen distal to the stent which did not respond to nitrate. Further AVE GFX 2.5 mm × 12 mm deployed in this area overlapping the first stent. Further distal segment showed tight narrowing with compromised distal flow. ACS MULTI-LINK® 2.5 mm × 25 mm stent deployed overlapping the AVE GFX. Still some narrowing of the distal end of this stent.

Antonio Bartorelli:

This complication is often due to distal dissection during stent deployment and may be related to direct injury of the atheromatous vessel wall caused by the distal edge of the stent or 'dog-boning' of the balloon outside the stent length. The best strategy to avoid a 'full metal jacket' with a suboptimal final result like this is to undersize the stent delivery system, especially in small vessels. The stent can always be post-dilated with a bigger balloon. Also in these cases, stent markers may avoid the edge dissection and occlusive flapping occur during intra-stent post-dilatation.

Case 5. Complications 1

64-year-old man. Ex-smoker; family history. 1992 Acute MI treated with streptokinase. 1992 PTCA to RCA with 3.0 mm Medtronic Wiktor® stent implantation. Recurrent pain 1996.

Catheter findings: Moderate LV with inferior hypokinesis; RCA unobstructed; LCA as shown.

Procedure: JL4 (8F) guide:
Circumflex: 0.014″ high torque floppy wire; 3.0 mm monorail balloon, Medtronic Wiktor 3.5 mm × 15 mm.

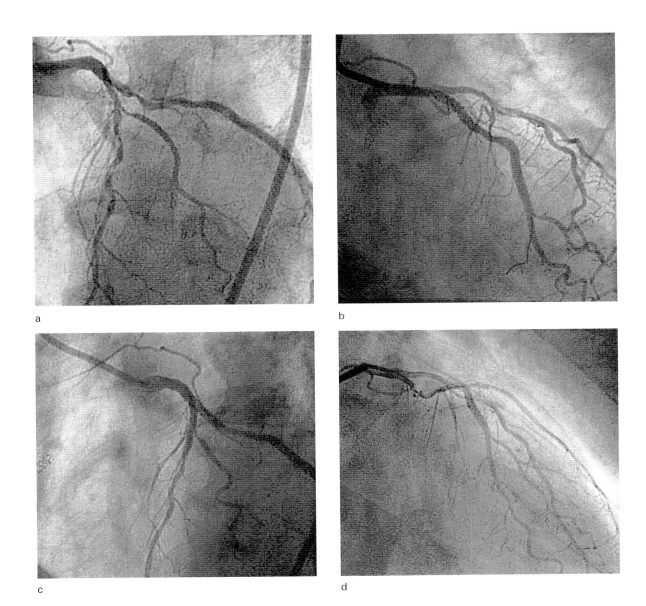

a

b

c

d

Figure 11.5
LCA angiogram. a) LAO view of difuse LAD disease, and significant proximal and mid-circumflex disease. b) RAO projection. c) Disrupted lesion in circumflex after proximal stent deployment. d) RAO view.

LAD: 0.014″ high torque floppy wire; 3.0-mm monorail balloon leading to local dissection. Attempted access with GFX 3.5 mm × 30 mm stent to LAD unsuccessful, and stent came off balloon in LMS.
Patient referred for urgent CABG with pain and anterior ST elevation.

Antonio Bartorelli:

The left anterior descending artery of this patient appears diffusely diseased, moderately tortuous and rigid. These are unfavourable characteristics for stent advancement and deployment. My suggested approach in these cases is to use guiding catheters with strong support and excellent coaxial alignment such as the Voda or the Extra back-up high-support wires, with the buddy wire technique (a second guidewire in the vessel to help maintain engagement and give extra support to the whole system) if necessary, and multiple short stent delivery systems with very low profile and good longitudinal flexibility.

An essential prerequisite for successfully stenting this type of lesion is to obtain adequate lesion pre-dilatation with a high-pressure balloon or debulking with rotational atherectomy in case of severe calcification. In this patient, the 30 mm long, 3.5 mm diameter GFX stent could not be completely advanced to cover the entire lesion and during attempted withdrawal slipped off the delivery balloon. If stent retrieval with grasping devices (snares, loops)[2] is unsuccessful, urgent CABG may be avoided with full deployment of the stent into the LMS and across the left circumflex ostium that, if not diseased, is rarely compromised by stent covering. After full stent expansion with a bigger balloon and achievement of a large stent lumen, the distal LAD disease may be subsequently treated by additional stenting.

Case 6. Complications 1

62-year-old man. Family history; high cholesterol. Stable angina.

Catheter findings: Minor inferior hypokinesis of LV; moderate lesion in mid-RCA; tight lesion in AVCx involving OM.

Procedure: JL4 8F guide; 0.014″ high torque floppy wires to both AVCx and OM. Both limbs pre-dilated with 3.0 mm monorail balloon. Cordis CrossFlex™ 3.0 mm × 25 mm stent in AVCx across OM origin and Cordis CrossFlex™ 3.0 mm × 15 mm stent through from AVCx into OM. Following deployment of the latter stent, dissection of the end into the distal OM with no flow. Despite extensive balloon inflations, no further stent could be passed into this part of the OM. OM therefore lost.

Antonio Bartorelli:

This is another example of stent edge dissection probably due to high-pressure deployment with a delivery balloon not matched with stent length and/or distal vessel dimension. Two approaches are available to avoid this complication: use of a delivery balloon exactly matched with stent length or stent deployment with an undersized delivery system at low pressure and subsequent high pressure post-dilatation with a short balloon with a 1 : 1 balloon/artery ratio. Once this complication occurs, recrossing an already deployed stent at the origin of a branch with an additional stent may be very difficult.

In this case protrusion into the parent vessel of the stent struts from the side-branch stent is the most likely reason for the procedural difficulty. Deep seating with long tip 6F guide catheters,[3] bending the stent into a gentle curve to steer it around protruding struts and forming a small bubble at the tip of the second delivery system to reduce the friction, may help in overcoming this problem.

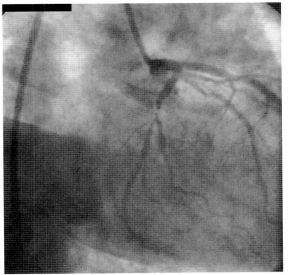

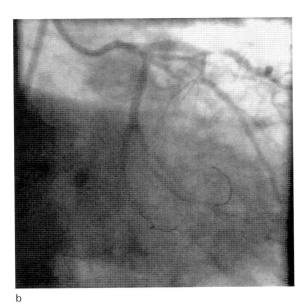

a

b

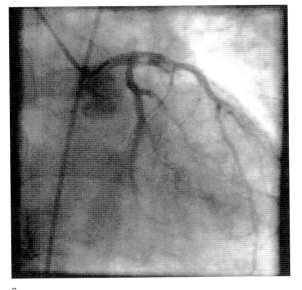

c

Figure 11.6
*LCA injection. a) Tight stenosis in circumflex
involving AVCx and OM. b) After stent in circumflex
flow to OM diminished. c) Result with OM lost.*

Case 7. Complications 1

66-year-old man. Ex-smoker. Inferior MI February 1998. Unstable angina March 1998.

Catheter findings: Moderate LV with inferior hypokinesis; complicated lesion in RCA.

Procedure: JR4 8F guide; 0.014″ high torque floppy wire; lesion pre-dilated with 3.0 mm monorail balloon. Cordis CrossFlex™ 4.0 mm × 15 mm stent deployed to 12 atm. Some waisting in stented area, therefore attempted to pass 4.0 mm Chubby™ balloon into middle of stent, but it would not go through.

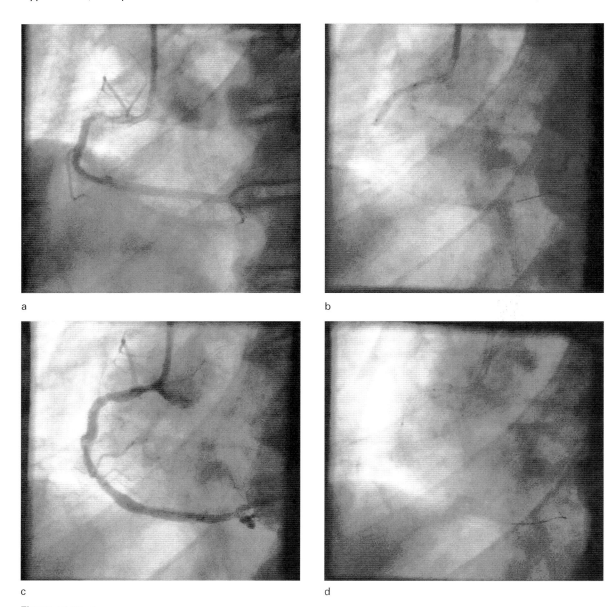

a

b

c

d

Figure 11.7a–g
RCA angiogram. a) Proximal significant disease. b) Proximal stent deployment. c) Result of primary procedure. d) Chubby™ balloon unable to cross.

Some disruption to outer curve of stent seen. Therefore, a further 4.0 mm × 25 mm Cordis CrossFlex™ deployed across the first stent to 14 atm.

Antonio Bartorelli:

Recrossing with a balloon catheter a stent already implanted in an angled segment of a large coronary vessel may pose a technical challenge. The first rule is not to use force. As in this case, the most likely result of excessive pushing will not be to cross the stent but instead cause it damage. Snagging of the balloon catheter distal tip against an incompletely apposed proximal stent strut is generally the cause of this problem.

A number of techniques may be applied to allow balloon catheter passage: changing the entry angle of the wire and balloon catheter by gently pushing forward or pulling out the guiding catheter, passing an additional wire, usually an extra support or stiff type (never forget to prolapse the wire J-tip during stent crossing), in order to further straighten the curved stented segment (buddy wire technique), and using a balloon-on-wire system, such as the ACE catheter, of larger diameter to completely appose the stent struts to the arterial wall.

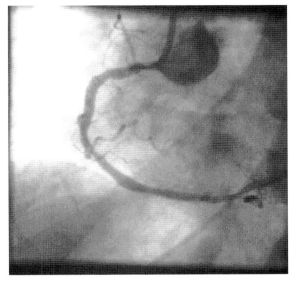

e

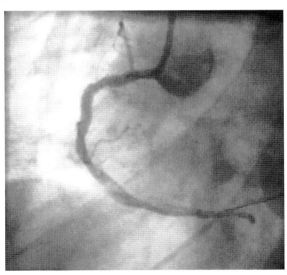

f

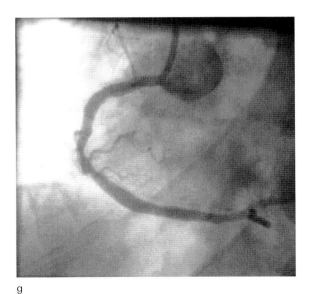

g

Figure 11.7 *continued*
e) Waist still present at proximal site of stenosis. f) Restented with second CrossFlex™. g) Post optimization result.

Case 8. Complications 1

64-year-old man. Smoker; family history. Limiting angina with ST depression in V3–V6 at ETT.

Catheter findings: Moderate LV; moderate stenosis in mid-RCA; LAD as shown.

Procedure: Amplatz left 2 8F guide; 0.014″ high torque floppy wire; 2.5 mm monorail balloon, then 3.0 mm × 15 mm ACS MULTI-LINK®. Intense spasm seen in LMS and circumflex with extensive ST segment elevation.

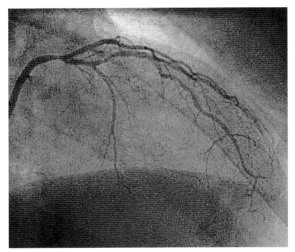

a

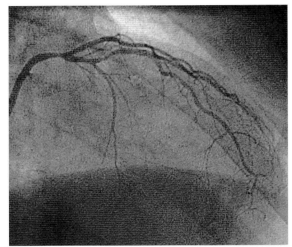

b

Figure 11.8
LCA angiogram. a) LAD stenosis just after septal perforator. b) After balloon dilatation. c) Result, good in stenosis, but intense spasm in LM.

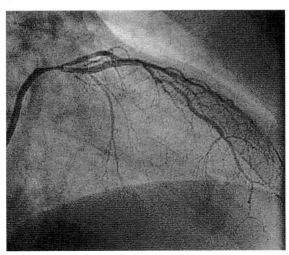

c

Case 9. Complications 1

60-year-old man. NIDDM, smoker; hypertensive. Unstable angina with anterior ECG changes.

Catheter findings: Good LV; discrete LAD disease; unobstructed RCA.

Procedure: JL4 8F guide; 0.014″ high torque floppy wire to LAD. 2.5 mm monorail balloon, then 3.5 mm × 25 mm ACS MULTI-LINK®. Intense LMS spasm during case with pain and ECG changes responding partially to intracoronary nitrate.

Antonio Bartorelli:

Cases 8 and 9 are taken together.

PTCA-induced coronary artery spasm has been reported in 1–5% of procedures.[4] Generally, it occurs at the site of the index lesion or in the distal epicardial vessel. The spasm generally responds to the intracoronary administration of nitroglycerine (200–300 µg). In cases refractory to repeated doses of nitroglycerine, intracoronary verapamil (100 µg/min up to 1.0–1.5 mg) or diltiazem (0.5–2.5 mg over > 1 min, total dose: 5–10 mg) may be used. If spasm resistant to pharmacological treatment occurs then prolonged low-pressure inflation (1–4 atm) with a balloon catheter matched 1 : 1 with the vessel size may be required for spasm resolution.

The intense spasm of the LMS observed in these two cases following LAD stenting could be related to mechanical irritation of the LMS due to deep seating of the guiding catheter. Guiding catheter withdrawal may resolve spasm in these cases. Partial removal of the guidewire, especially if a stiff type has been used, until only the soft distal tip traverses the affected segment, could be another approach to reduce mechanical irritation.[5] However, refractory spasm should always raise the suspicion of superimposed coronary dissection and thrombus. Multiple angiographic views and intravascular ultrasound should always be used to clarify the pathophysiology of the lumen narrowing and to guide management of refractory spasm.

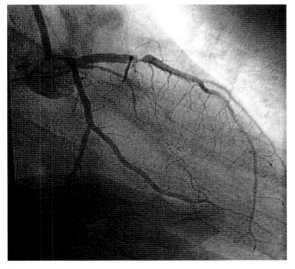

a

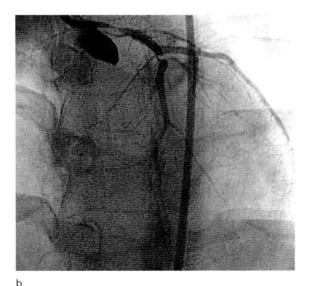

b

Figure 11.9a–d
LCA angiogram. a) Severe mid-LAD short lesion, LM appears small. b) Intense LM spasm, prior to LAD dilatation.

continued

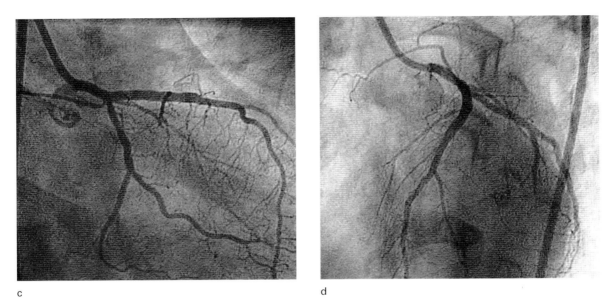

c   d

Figure 11.9 *continued*
c) After stent deployment and intracoronary NTG. d) LAO view of result in LAD, and relief of spasm.

Case 10. Complications 1

55-year-old man. High cholesterol; ex-smoker. Limiting exertional angina. Previous inferior MI, 1995.

Catheter findings: LV: minor inferior hypokinesis; unobstructed LAD; 80% stenosis in circumflex; tight RCA stenosis in mid-vessel.

Procedure: JR4 8F; 0.014″ high torque floppy wire backed up with 3.0 mm over-the-wire balloon. Stented using a 3.5 mm × 30 mm AVE GFX. Stent thrombosis that evening. Disobliterated with 0.014″ high torque floppy wire and 3.0 mm balloon. IVUS demonstrated dissection proximal to the stent. Proximal vessel stented using 4.0 mm × 15 mm ACS MULTI-LINK®. Obvious discrete clot seen at end. Abciximab (ReoPro®). Clot still present in vessel 3 days later at redo angiogram.

Antonio Bartorelli:

Small stent edge dissections may be invisible at final angiographic control after stent implantation, but may become subocclusive in the hours following intervention, favouring early subacute thrombosis as demonstrated in this case. When a 3.5 mm × 30 mm stent thromboses, a substantial amount of fresh thrombus accumulates into the stent lumen and creates several treatment challenges. My preferred management of these particular cases is pharmacological therapy with ReoPro®, which has been demonstrated to have a dissolution effect on platelet-rich thrombus, followed by placement of a distal protection device to avoid distal embolization of fresh clot during vessel recanalization. The residual thrombus shown at repeat angiogram 3 days later may represent a nidus for further re-thrombosis and should be addressed. In my experience, ultrasound thrombolysis may help both to reduce the clot burden and to lyse the residual thrombosis still present in the vessel lumen.[6]

Figure 11.10
RCA angiogram. a) Angiogram 6 hours after successful stenting of mid-RCA lesion (ReoPro® not given at primary procedure). b) Appearance after passage of guidewire. Flow delineates distal appearance of thrombus. ReoPro® given after proximal stent for dissection confirmed by IVUS. c) 3 days later clot still visible in distal vessel.

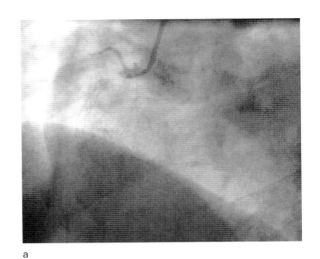

a

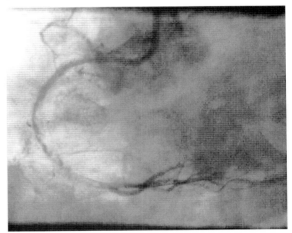

b

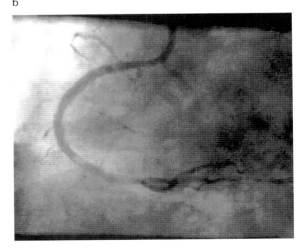

c

References

1. Laird JR, Popma JJ, Knopf WD, et al. Angiographic and procedural outcome after coronary angioplasty in high-risk subsets using a decremental diameter (tapered) balloon catheter. Am J Cardiol 1996;77:561–568.
2. Foster-Smith KW, Garrat KN, Higaro ST, Holmes DR. Retrieval techniques for managing flexible intracoronary stent misplacement. Cathet Cardiovasc Diagn 1993;30:63–68.
3. Bartorelli AL, Lavarra F, Trabattoni D, et al. Successful stent delivery with deep seating of 6 French guiding catheter in difficult coronary anatomy. Cathet Cardiovasc Intervent 1999;48: 279–284.
4. Cowley M, Dorros G, Kelsey S, et al. Acute coronary events associated with percutaneous transluminal coronary angioplasty. Am J Cardiol 1984;53:12C–16C.
5. Tenaglia AN, Tcheng JE, Phillips HR, Stack RS. Creation of pseudo narrowing during coronary angioplasty. Am J Cardiol 1991;67:658–659.
6. Rosenchein U, Gaul G, Erbel R, et al. Percutaneous transluminal therapy of occluded saphenous vein grafts: can the challenge be met with ultrasound thrombolysis? Circulation 1999;99:26–29.

12
Complications 2 – dissections

The occurrence of vessel dissection is often nowadays taken as no more than confirmation that the pre-dilatation balloon has been effective. Nevertheless, dissection can be unpredictable and potentially disastrous. The interventionist tends to build up a wide range of technical skills that he or she draws from to respond appropriately to these circumstances. The following cases help to illustrate some of these.

Comment is provided by **Hans Bonnier** and **Chaim Lotan**.

Case 1. Complications 2

48-year-old woman. Family history. Limiting angina.

Catheter findings: Good LV; unobstructed LCA; discrete lesion in RCA.

Procedure: JR4 8F; 0.014″ high torque floppy wire; single inflation with 2.5 mm monorail balloon lead to extensive dissection backwards and forwards with inferior ST elevation and pain. 2 ACS MULTI-LINK® stents deployed from ostium to distal vessel as follows: (a) ACS MULTI-LINK® 3.0 mm × 35 mm; (b) ACS MULTI-LINK® 3.0 mm × 25 mm.

Hans Bonnier:

One of the most important issues in interventional cardiology is choosing the correct guiding catheter. The Judkins right tip often points to the inferior luminal surface of the vessel. This sometimes makes vessel access difficult because of a very sharp angle and this can present extra difficulty for stenting. For this reason I created the Bonnier-right (Fig. 12.1e), for which I changed the angle of the catheter and also made a more smooth curve. In 95% of all cases it creates a straightforward channel into the vessel. In this particular case it would have been of great help.

Another issue is how long the balloon should be to dilate this lesion. The lesion looks a little bit hazy and perhaps contains thrombus. We would therefore choose to start with abciximab some hours before the procedure and probably directly stent the lesion using a stent of ≤ 15 mm (e.g. ACS MULTI-LINK® 3.0 mm RX Duet™, or Biotronik TENAX™ 15 mm × 3.0 mm). In this case with this extensive dissection backwards and forwards, the solution is to implant one long stent such as a monorail Magic Wallstent® or 2 ACS MULTI-LINK® stents. With the latter choice, the first should be placed distal to the dissection and the second at the proximal end. This will lead to a nice result but we should keep in mind the fact that the longer the metal jacket the higher the rate of restenosis.[1–3]

Chaim Lotan:

A spiral dissection of the RCA is one of the most dreadful nightmares of the interventional cardiologist. It can change a discrete 'innocent' lesion into a rapid unzipping of the artery with abrupt occlusion and haemodynamic compromise. In response to this, quick inflation of a long balloon, with small diameter (2.0 mm or 2.5 mm), can be attempted and may usually restore some flow, even temporarily. This may also ensure that a

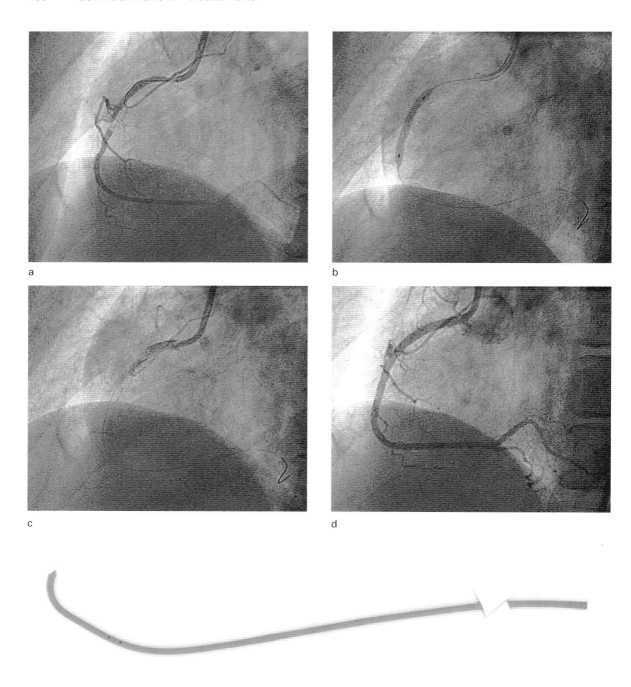

Figure 12.1
RCA angiogram. a) Discrete lesion in mid-RCA immediately after RV branch. b) Balloon dilatation with 2.5 mm balloon. c) Extensive dissection. d) Result after 2 stents. e) Bonnier-right guide catheter.

stent can be safely deployed. By contrast, the use of an 'adequately sized' balloon may exacerbate the dissection. The early administration of IIb/IIIa inhibitors is very important, as thrombus starts to form immediately. Abciximab is a good option, but in cases where CABG is considered, the use of tirofiban or eptafibatide may be preferable.

If quick balloon inflations do restore some flow in the artery and the entire length of the dissection can be appreciated, including the proximal and distal ends, two long flexible stents (either ACS MULTI-LINK® or AVE 670) should be deployed. If there is some flow in the artery and the distal end of the dissection can adequately be seen, the distal end should be stented first, in order to secure the distal end and prevent distal propagation. This may also alleviate the need for passing a long stent through a proximally deployed stent. However, in cases where no flow exists in the artery, the proximal stent should be deployed first, and stenting should continue according to the angiographic findings.

Tips

It is extremely important to secure the guidewire distally and be very careful with guidewire manipulations. Losing the wire position can be a big problem as it is very difficult in these cases to restore wire position and assure that the wire is in a true lumen and not in a false lumen, in which case stenting might lead to disaster. Thus, only very flexible stents should be used without too much force. In tortuous arteries, or in those cases where extra support is needed, it is wise to replace the wire with a 'stent supporting wire' such as the ACS-BMW or even the Schneider Hannibal™. This can be done by placing an over-the-wire balloon or the multi-function probing system from Schneider over the in-situ guidewire, advancing the balloon or sheath to the distal vessel, and then replacing the guidewire with the stiffer wire; this technique avoids losing the distal guidewire position. The extra time spent undertaking this procedure could save a lot of time and aggravation later.

Case 2. Complications 2

69-year-old woman. Ex-smoker; high cholesterol. Acute inferior MI treated with streptokinase. Thirty days later, further admission with acute pain and lateral T changes.

Catheter findings: Moderate LV with inferior hypokinesis; tight stenosis in proximal circumflex; occluded RCA and unobstructed LAD.

Procedure: JL4 8F; 0.014″ high torque floppy wire. Pre-dilatation with 3.0 mm monorail balloon, then Cordis CrossFlex™ 3.5 mm × 15 mm stent. Dissection seen at distal end of stent at bifurcation between AV circumflex and OM. Further 3.0 mm × 15 mm Cordis CrossFlex™ deployed overlapping first stent distally, giving good OM flow, but compromised flow down AVCx due to a large dissection.

Hans Bonnier:

Also in this case the choice of the correct guiding catheter is an important one. First, for the circumflex an Amplatz catheter gives more back-up support than the Judkins left in most cases. Another important issue is: should we use an 8F or 6F catheter? Nowadays in all cases (except when we use Rotablator, directional coronary atherectomy, transluminal extraction atherectomy or excimer laser coronary angioplasty and IVUS) we use 6F guiding catheters, which lead to fewer dissections. All new stent designs are 6F compatible.

In this particular case, you have to pre-dilate and try to get a stent-like result, because stenting the circumflex or dilating only with a balloon

makes no big difference in the long term according to BENESTENT II.[4] Having implanted a Cordis CrossFlex™ stent in this case and created a dissection distal to the stent, we would question whether or not the CrossFlex™ is the best stent for this lesion? In this case I would use a 20 mm Wiktor®-I 3.5 mm stent, which is probably the most flexible stent for these curves.

In this case where another Cordis CrossFlex™ stent was implanted it proved impossible to access a wire in the AVCx. Maybe the only solution for this problem is the use of Abciximab to prevent thrombosis. At least if the less important limb closes, the long-term outcome will probably not be less favourable.[5]

Chaim Lotan:

Dissection at the stent edges (usually at the distal end) is quite a common but under-reported phenomenon. This complication can be seen particularly with high-pressure deployment and occurs in our experience in about 10–20% of cases (depending on the type of stent and the deployment balloon). It is the main reason for additional stent deployment after stenting.

The type of treatment is dependent upon the flow disturbance. Very small dissection (type a) can be left untouched or treated with IIb/IIIa inhibitors. However, in these cases, the operator should wait 10–15 minutes for a final angiogram before leaving the room. In the case of large dissections (>type b) an additional stent is usually necessary. Care should be taken to select a short, flexible stent that should be deployed with minimal overlap over the first stent with moderate pressure (~10 atm). The balloon should then be withdrawn a few

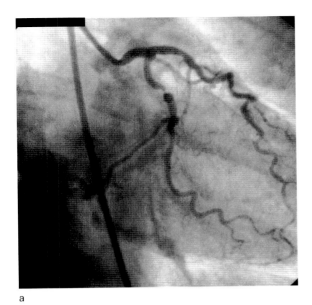

a

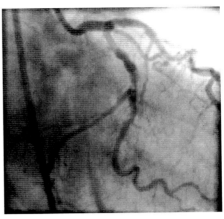

b

Figure 12.2
LCA angiogram. a) Tight circumflex stenosis. b) After first stent deployment waist still present at lesion site and disruption seen at origin of OM and AVCx.

millimetres, well into the first stent, and the point of stent overlap should be inflated with higher pressure (~14–16 atm), to assure optimal deployment.

Tips

The judgment about treatment strategies for jeopardized or 'jailed' branches is dependent upon their relative importance. In the current case, the jeopardized AVCx groove artery is usually of marginal importance and thus no additional step should be taken. However, if significant ischaemic changes occur, attempts should be made to cross out of the side of the stent into the side branch. In my view, given the angulations of the jailed branch, a stiff tip 'standard' wire with a large 'J', or an ACE fixed wire system (Scimed, Boston Scientific) should be tried. The use of IIb/IIIa inhibitors may help to preserve flow in important side branches.

Case 3. Complications 2

51-year-old man. Ex-smoker; high cholesterol. CABG surgery 1995 (LIMA to LAD; vein grafts to OM, intermediate and diagonal). Presented with unstable angina.

Catheter findings: LV function moderate; RCA as shown. All grafts patent.

Procedure: Amplatz left 2 8F guide; 0.014″ high torque floppy wire crossed lesion backed up by 2.0 mm over-the-wire balloon. Dilatation at line of occlusion with 3.0 mm monorail balloon. Large dissection seen from guide catheter inwards and staining back into coronary sinus.

Hans Bonnier:

The guiding chosen in this case is reasonable, but 8F may not be the best choice. The choice of a 2.0 mm over-the-wire balloon as back up support is good, but why use a 3.0 mm monorail balloon afterwards to dilate the vessel? The 2.0 mm Bandit balloon reaches 2.4 mm with high pressure and that is enough to stent this lesion directly. Good stent choices would be the Cordis MiniCrown, the Boston Scientific NIR™, the ACS MULTI-LINK RX Duet™ or the Biotronik TENAX™. But in this case with a huge dissection at the beginning of the right and probably to the end of the stenosis, I would use a monorail Wallstent® of 50 mm (and pray to God that after I placed that stent from the beginning of the right coronary artery to the distal part after the stenosis that the artery is fine!). Otherwise there is only one solution: send the patient to the surgery department, for a minimally invasive procedure without a pump.

If the right is small and the Wallstent® did not have any effect, doing nothing is also a possible solution which will result in a small inferior wall infarction. What the correct solution is, is not always clear. Abciximab will not result in a better outcome in this case.

Chaim Lotan:

Careful intubation and guide-catheter manipulation in 'shepherd's crook' take-off of the RCA is extremely important. If support is needed an Amplatz Right or even an Amplatz Lt-2 are a good choice, but should be handled with extra care. It is better to choose softer tips and smaller guiding catheters (6F instead of 8F).

In case of a significant ostial dissection caused by the guide catheter, as seen in this case, prompt stenting of the ostium should be performed. A flexible stent with good radial support and coverage should be chosen. The optimal length is 15–18 mm as shorter stents are more difficult to place in the ostium when the guide catheter is outside the ostium, and longer stents might have trackability problems in this anatomy. The stent should not protrude out of the ostium more than 1–2 mm in order not to interfere with future intubation of the ostium. After deployment of the stent the balloon should be partly withdrawn and inflated with higher pressure to form a 'funnel shape' which may facilitate future guide catheter insertion.

The long-term prognosis of these ostial dissections is usually good, even if they extend into the sinus. Even though the angiographic appearance might be worrisome, these dissections rarely lead to ostial occlusion (after stenting of the ostium) and rarely propagate proximally, so bail-out to CABG will not be necessary in the majority of cases and should be performed only if flow cannot be restored in the more distal part of the artery.

In our judgement the use of IIb/IIIa inhibitors in such a case is relatively contraindicated as we like to have the false channel caused by the dissection thrombose off. Nevertheless, if the results of the PCI in the RCA are less than satisfactory, small-molecule, short-acting IIb/IIIa inhibitors can be used with caution.

Tips

With such a tortuous anatomy, the guidewire should be replaced with a stiffer wire that will provide the additional support needed to continue the treatment and stenting of the mid-RCA lesion. Care should be taken to optimally pre-dilate the lesion before further stenting and to use a flexible and trackable stent (the AVE 670 for example).

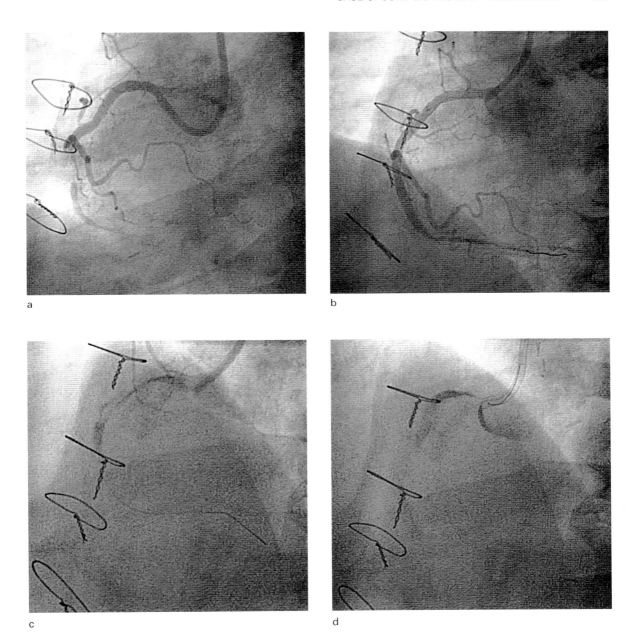

Figure 12.3
RCA angiogram. a) Upward pointing take-off of RCA and mid-RCA tight stenosis are seen. b) Initial satisfactory result after small balloon dilatation. c) Dissection seen at lesion site and proximally. d) Vessel occluded with proximal staining on RCA and sinus.

Case 4. Complications 2

51-year-old man. Ex-smoker; hypercholesterol-aemia; family history. Stable, limiting angina.

Catheter findings: Good LV; long segment of LAD disease; significant stenosis in proximal area of first diagonal branch; unobstructed circumflex; moderate lesion in mid-RCA.

Procedure: JL4 8F guide; 0.014″ high torque floppy wire. Segment of LAD disease pre-dilated with 3.0 mm monorail balloon. Cordis CrossFlex™ 3.0 mm × 25 mm stent passed into this segment with great difficulty, requiring very aggressive guide catheter engagement. Dissection seen in proximal LAD and left main stem. Dissected area stented with ACS MULTI-LINK® 3.5 mm × 25 mm. Abciximab (ReoPro®) given.

Hans Bonnier:

The price you pay for placing a stent in the LAD, although the segment is pre-dilated with a balloon, can be high. First of all you should ask yourself what to do with the significant stenosis in the proximal area of the first diagonal branch? I would start with this vessel and examine very carefully from different angles to see whether the vessel is well treated. If this is not the case a small stent can be the solution, but it should be placed very precisely only in the diagonal.

The indication for placing a stent in the long diseased LAD segment is clear, but perhaps the use of a slotted tube stent is better than a coil stent in this segment. Personally I mainly use slotted tube stents in the proximal LAD. Nevertheless, after implanting the Cordis CrossFlex™ there is a dissection caused by the aggressive use of the 8F guiding catheter. The strategy of implanting an ACS MULTI-LINK® and giving abciximab is a good one. In the past year stenting of the left main is a topic that has been very highly placed on the agenda of every inter-ventional congress. A lot of data are available and it seems feasible and encouraging,[6,7] although there are no studies available where a part of the left main is stented after dissections. The result after stenting the dissection is nice and I would send the patient home 1 day after ending the abciximab administration.

Chaim Lotan:

Ostial LAD and main stem dissection due to aggressive guide catheter manipulation are among the common nightmares of the interven-tional cardiologist. The first rule to deal with such complications is to avoid them: care (and experience...) is needed to stay away from aggressive manipulation of a guiding catheter with a long stent in a tortuous artery.

Once a dissection has occurred, stenting of the proximal/ostial LAD should be performed using a short stent with high radio-opacity (like the NIR™ Royal from Boston Scientific), to enable precise deployment. In cases where there is a minor dissection of the superior part of the main stem, a more conservative approach can be taken. However, if the dissection largely involves the main stem, with proximal progression towards the ostium (very rare), stenting of the left main should be considered and performed if the anatomy is suitable (in other words, if there is enough length to the left main to allow stenting without interfering with the ostium of the LCX).

Any interference with the flow to the LCX (either before or after stenting) should indicate the need for bailout CABG, and therefore a IIb/IIIa should not be given. In all other cases, the use of a IIb/IIIa is justified. The guidewire should be pulled out only after repeated injections (after 20–30 minutes) fail to demonstrate any flow disturbances or filling defects in the entire proximal left system.

The length of the hospital stay is a real dilemma and is largely dependent upon the course of the PCI, the need for IABP, the use of IIb/IIIa's and the final result. It should not be too short, as there is a need to ensure good recov-ery of the patient and the operator, but on the other hand as admission that is too long is not 'healthy' for the patient. Thus, a few extra days in hospital with some kind of a challenging test (ETT if appropriate or myocardial perfusion scan) seems reasonable.

Tips

A long tortuous/calcified lesion in the proximal LAD is among the known 'painful' lesions that may herald the upcoming complication. Thus, such lesions should be treated with 'respect'. Attempts should be made to maximize pre-dilation of the entire segment and properly

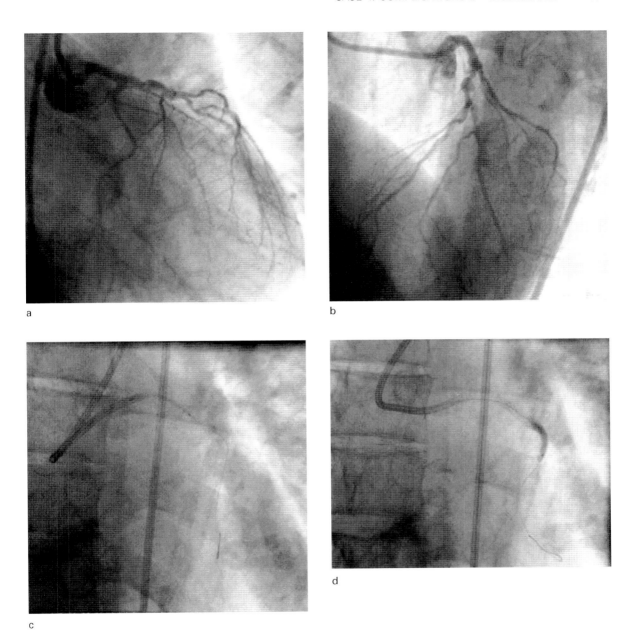

Figure 12.4a–i
LCA angiogram. a) Tight proximal LAD stenosis and mid-LAD stenosis in RAO. b) As above in LAO. c) Deep guide catheter engagement to back-up balloon advancement. d) Balloon inflated in mid-LAO.

continued

prepare the 'bed' for the stent. It is also wise to use an extra-support guidewire in order to facilitate stent delivery and minimize 'deep throating' of the guiding catheter.

In addition, short stents should be used for the most problematic parts of the lesion (either non-compliant or recoil is seen), rather then trying to cover the entire lesion with very long stents.

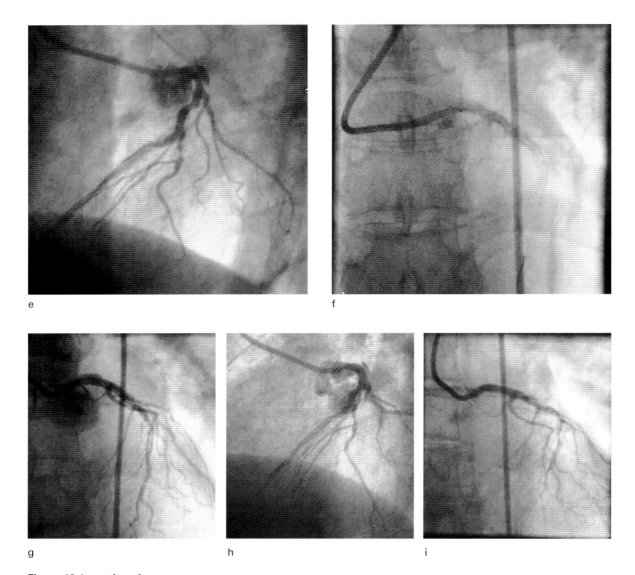

Figure 12.4 *continued*
e) Disrupted LM. f) Stent deployment in LM. g) Result of LM stent. h) Good LM appearance, but staining persistent outside lumen channel. i) Result.

Case 5. Complications 2

79-year-old woman. Ex-smoker; hypertension. History of CVA; carotid Doppler examinations showing critical stenosis at origin of right internal carotid artery and complete occlusion in left internal carotid. Presented with unstable angina. LBBB on ECG.

Catheter findings: Significant LV impairment with significant stenoses in LAD and circumflex vessels. Turned down for CABG.

Procedure: Amplatz left 2 guide 8F, 0.014″ high torque floppy wire to LAD. Lesion pre-dilated and then stented with 3.5 mm × 15 mm Cordis CrossFlex™ without difficulty. Then wire passed into circumflex, but LMS dissection noted off end of guide in LMS. Despite attempts at stenting of the LMS, cardiac arrest occurred and resuscitation unsuccessful.

Hans Bonnier:

This is a typical case, which fortunately does not occur every day at the catheterization laboratory.

This concerns an old woman, turned down for CABG, who had typical unstable angina symptoms and disease in all arteries.

There are two stenoses in the left coronary artery and the interventional cardiologist is thinking that the case is easy to perform. The choice of the guiding catheter is questionable. Perhaps a U-shaped guider or a normal left Judkins was a better choice and a 6F catheter instead of 8F should also have lowered the risk of complications. To pre-dilate and stent the lesions is a good idea, but choosing the right stent for these lesions is difficult and contentious. In the LAD the choice of a Cordis CrossFlex™ may have been reasonable. I would not have used the Cordis Crossflex™ LC, the Medtronic beStent™ or the Boston Scientific NIR™ stent in either this vessel or in the circumflex, because the lesion is on a bend, a coiled stent (such as the Medtronic Wiktor®-I or Cordis CrossFlex™) in this type of lesion is a better solution.

Unfortunately, in this case a left main dissection occurred and, despite the attempt to stent this dissection, there was a cardiac arrest and resuscitation was unsuccessful.

The cause of the dissection could be the guiding catheter and this is the reason that I would not use this type of guide if treating both the LAD and the circumflex. An ACS MULTI-LINK RX DUET™ or Cordis MiniCrown stent would probably have been the best choice in this case to stent the left main but unfortunately the case turned out in the wrong direction.

Chaim Lotan:

Patients turned down for CABG comprise usually a very high-risk group for PCI. It is always important to remember that bad cases remain bad cases. This relatively elderly female patient with significant carotid stenosis, impairment of LV function and significant lesions in extremely tortuous LAD and circumflex arteries is definitely a high-risk patient.

In such patients, other conservative treatment alternatives should be thoroughly discussed:

- Let's give the patient a chance to stabilize.
- Consider off-bypass LIMA to the LAD, and delayed treatment of the circumflex.
- PCI to the most severe lesion (the lesion judged to be responsible for the patient's symptoms).

The use of the Amplatz guiding catheter provides extra support, especially with the current anatomy, but the drawbacks of this guiding should be noted and its handling should be performed with extra care. Prophylactic insertion of IABP (or at least another femoral sheath) in such patients is highly advisable, as haemodynamic deterioration in such a case can be very quick because of the lack of myocardial reserve.

Tips

When attempting to do a complex PCI in very complex anatomy, patients should be *pre-treated* with IIb/IIIa inhibitors. Secondly, when attempting to dilate the proximal segments of the LAD and LCX, it might be useful to leave the wire in the LAD after the dilatation and approach the lesion in the LCX with a second wire.

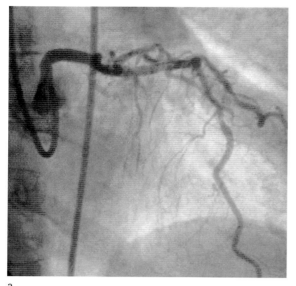

a

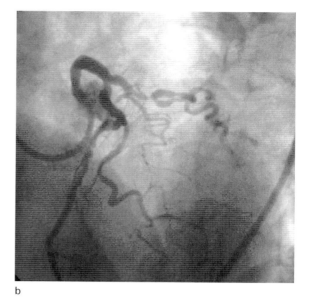

b

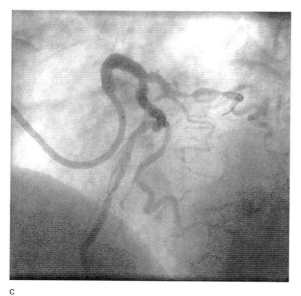

c

Figure 12.5a–f
*LCA angiogram. a) Mid and distal LAD lesions seen.
b) LAD disease and circumflex significant stenoses
seen. c) Proximal LAD stented.*

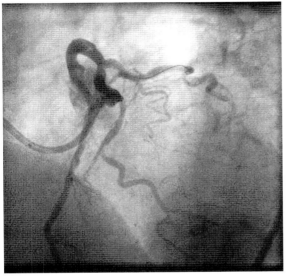

d

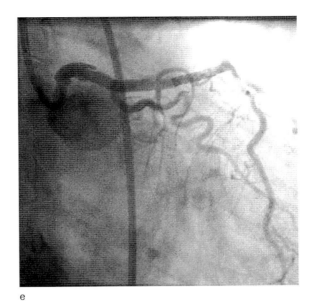

e

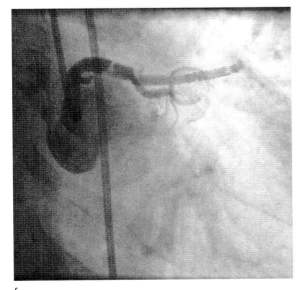

f

Figure 12.5 *continued*
d) Wire in circumflex but not advanced. e) LM dissected. f) Poor flow to circumflex and distal run-off from LAD stent poor.

References

1. Hamasaki N, et al. Influence of lesion length on late angiographic outcome and restenotic process after successful implantation. JACC 1997; 29 (suppl A):239A(abstract).

2. Pemerantsev E, et al. Angiographic predictors of restenosis after optimal coronary stent deployment. Circulation 1997;96(suppl):I–473 (abstract).

3. Kobayashi Y, et al. The length of the stented segment is an independent predictor of restenosis. JACC 1998;31(Suppl):366A(abstract).

4. Serruys P, et al. Effectiveness, cost and cost effectiveness of strategy of elective heparin-coated stenting compared with balloon angioplasty in selected patients with coronary artery disease: The Benestent II Study. Lancet 1998;352:673–681.

5. Grenadier E, et al. Coronary artery side-branch jailing after stent deployment: acute and long-term results. Int J Cardiovasc Intervent 1999;2(Suppl 2):11.

6. Park SJ, et al. Stenting of unprotected left main coronary artery stenoses: immediate and late outcome. JACC 1998;31:37–42.

7. Ellis SG, et al. Contemporary percutaneous treatment of unprotected left main stenosis—a preliminary report of the ULTIMA registry. Circulation 1996;94(Suppl):1–671.

13
Stent thrombosis

Thrombosis is an unusual complication after stent placement these days with the routine use of anti-platelet therapies. Often thrombosis occurs on the basis of dissection (sometimes unseen) proximal or distal to the stent, perhaps caused by the protruding shoulders of the balloon. Infrequently it is associated with a poorly deployed stent, again unseen. Poor run-off downstream to the stent can contribute to slow flow and then thrombosis. Likewise the patient can have a propensity to thrombosis which is not overcome by our current therapeutic manoeuvres.

General considerations when thrombosis occurs after stent placement:

- Abciximab (ReoPro®): when to start it?... whilst waiting for the laboratory to open?
- Which wire should we lead with.... Backed up or not?
- Are there techniques with the guidewire for avoiding stent struts and to test whether we are wholly within the stent lumen?
- How do we size the balloon?
- Is there a place for clot removal or distal protection devices?

Nick Curzen comments on the cases and provides the following preamble.

The rate of stent thrombosis has fallen drastically as a direct result of an improved understanding of the key role of platelet activation and aggregation in the pathophysiological sequence that produces it. The reduction in incidence to no more than 1% is one of the key reasons that some centres are now able to perform coronary stent procedures on a day-case basis.

The introduction of the anti-platelet regimen of aspirin plus ticlopidine[1] was a landmark in the evolution of coronary stenting. The subsequent switch to the less toxic clopidogrel in place of ticlopidine[2] represents a further significant refinement that has not only improved patient safety but also rendered obsolete the time-consuming and costly monitoring that used to be necessary.[3] Nevertheless, it is probably also true that such effective regimes for the inhibition of platelet aggregation mask both our need and desire to understand *why* the stent thrombosis phenomenon occurs in some patients.

The following cases raise this and the related issues of investigation and management of this complication. The most important of these questions can be summarized as follows:

- Why did the thrombosis occur?
- How much investigation does this require? Angiography only or with IVUS?
- Does thrombolysis help?
- Which wire?
- Over-the-wire balloon?

Case 1. Stent thrombosis

55-year-old man. Ex-smoker. Inferior MI 1995. Stable, limiting angina.

Catheter findings: LV function good overall, with mild inferior hypokinesis; long tight lesion in dominant RCA; LCA unobstructed.

Procedure: JR4 8F guide; 0.014″ high torque floppy wire; 3.0 mm monorail balloon; 3.5 mm × 30 mm GFX stent to 10 atm. Good angiographic result. 6 hours later, developed pain with inferior ST elevation. Angiogram as shown. Disobliteration with 0.014″ high torque floppy wire and 3.0 mm over-the-wire balloon, with thrombus seen in vessel. IVUS demon-

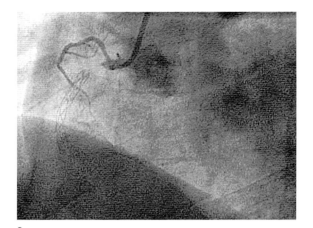

a

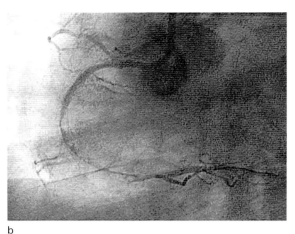

b

Figure 13.1
RCA angiogram. a) 6 hours after satisfactory angioplasty and stent procedure. Vessel occluded proximal to stent. b) Appearance after passage of curve. c) Balloon inflation throughout vessel led to visualization of clot in mid/distal portion of RCA.

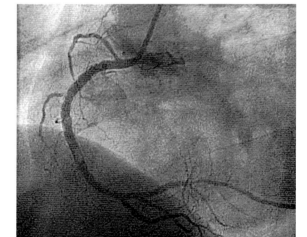

c

strated dissection off the proximal end of the stent; 4.0 mm × 15 mm ACS MULTI-LINK® overlapping first stent. Abciximab (ReoPro®) bolus and infusion.

Nick Curzen:

In this case a long stent has been deployed at only 10 atm. There seems to be general consensus that, particularly in the right coronary artery, it is important not to underestimate the target luminal diameter. In the cases where the vessel appears to have a diameter between 3.0 mm and 3.5 mm, the tendency is therefore to choose the larger stent. In this case, the 3.5 mm stent was deployed and stent thrombosis occurred. IVUS has been employed to good effect in determining that the underlying cause for the thrombosis was probably a dissection off the proximal end of the stent. This knowledge has clearly affected the clinical management, because on the strength of this knowledge a more proximal stent is deployed to cover the flap. This raises an interesting question: is IVUS necessary in order to investigate and manage stent thrombosis in an optimal fashion? The answer is a matter for debate. On the one hand this case illustrates that without IVUS the possible causal lesion would not necessarily have been identified and treated appropriately. On the other hand, stent thrombosis is effectively treated in catheter laboratories in which IVUS is not available. Such treatment is based upon the robust strategy that the top priority must be given to reopening the vessel mechanically and disrupting the thrombus. Subsequent therapy after this primary objective has been achieved is then determined by angiographic appearances alone.

What seems incontrovertible is that, the thrombus having been disrupted mechanically, the administration of abciximab provides the pharmacological means for encouraging the clot to break down and removing the potential for it to reform by inhibiting platelet aggregation. The IIb/IIIa inhibitor seems especially well suited to this task. By contrast, the experience seems to be that thrombolysis is a less effective therapy for this particular brand of acute MI than it is in de novo myocardial infarction. The temptation to administer some or all of the abciximab bolus into the coronary is probably not very logical but is one that I nevertheless find impossible to resist! The use of IIb/IIIa inhibitors significantly reduces the chance of angiographically unseen dissections causing recurrent problems even when they are left unstented.

The ideal treatment strategy for stent thrombosis (regardless of whether the patient (a) re-presents to the Emergency department after having gone home; or (b) experiences the thrombosis whilst still in hospital) would therefore be as shown in Fig. 13.1d.

The other interesting aspect of this case is that the initial strategy, post-thrombosis, was to use an over-the-wire balloon. This was in order to provide extra support to the wire as it is advanced through the long stented segment. There should appropriately be some concern about avoiding advancing the wire behind or between the stent struts. The danger of this is

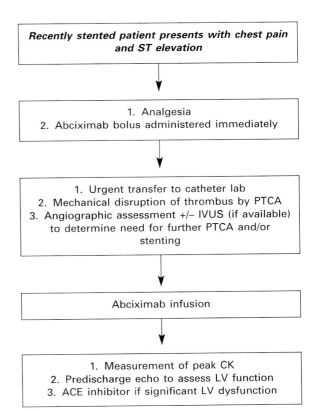

Figure 13.1d
Ideal treatment of stent thrombosis? (regardless of the site of presentation)

very real because often the vessel is still occluded when the wire makes this journey and is therefore being advanced blindly. Passage of the over-the-wire balloon a few millimetres behind the leading tip of the wire is one strategy to minimize the risk of this happening. Regardless of the type of balloon used in such circumstances, a feeling of resistance to the advance of the balloon should ring alarm bells that the wire has gone behind one or more stent struts. If there is doubt, the safest thing is probably to rewire.

Case 2. Stent thrombosis

61-year-old man. High cholesterol; NIDDM. Stable angina. Angioplasty 3 days previously with two 3.5 mm × 18 mm AVE GFX stents in the LAD.

Presentation with anterior ST elevation and pain.

Procedure: JL4 8F guide; 0.014″ high torque intermediate wire with 3.5 mm monorail balloon. Extensive dilatation in stents and between. Further Cordis CrossFlex™ 3.0 mm × 15 mm deployed overlapping distal end of lower stent where a dissection could be seen. Abciximab (ReoPro®) given.

Nick Curzen:

It again appears that the culprit lesion responsible for this thrombosis is an edge dissection. This time a slightly stiffer wire is used to disobliterate the vessel. I favour this type of wire as its increased stiffness allows it a greater chance of finding a way through the thrombus. On the other hand, stiffer wires are more likely to pick up stent struts or intimal flaps, especially in this 'blind' situation. After the wire has passed through into the distal vessel it is a good idea to push the deflated balloon through the occlusion into the vessel beyond the stent in order to check that no stent strut has been picked up, before going back to dilate. The aim of the balloon dilatations that are then performed is not completely clear. Obviously the primary aim is to disrupt the thrombus so that the IIb/IIIa inhibitor can gain adequate access. This could be achieved with a smaller-diameter balloon than the stent or a balloon of the same diameter at low pressure. Usually, however, the balloon chosen is of the same diameter as the stent and is then inflated to high pressure. What is the logic of this? Is there evidence that stent thrombosis occurs because stents are not fully deployed? Is there any evidence that higher inflation pressures make the thrombus dissolution more efficient? If the balloon is not contained completely within the stent then presumably there is a chance of exacerbating or creating dissection at this location? My current strategy is therefore to use a low pressure inflation with a reference diameter-sized balloon within the stent to

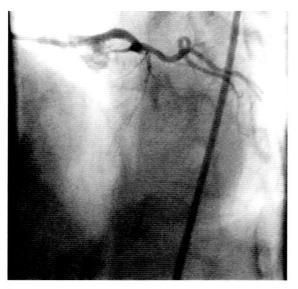

a

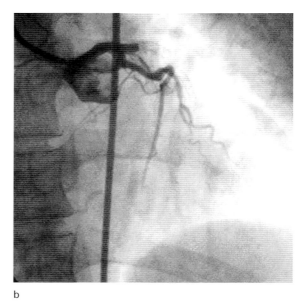

b

Figure 13.2a–e
LCA angiogram. a) Total occlusion of LAD, in stent. b) Stent seen with 'cut-off' LAD, an appearance often consistent with thrombosis.

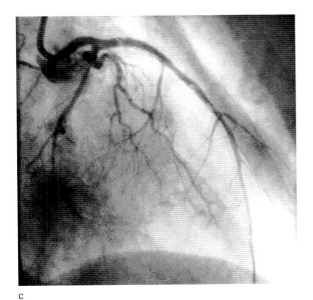

c

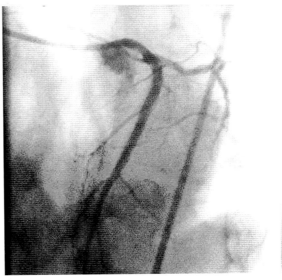

d

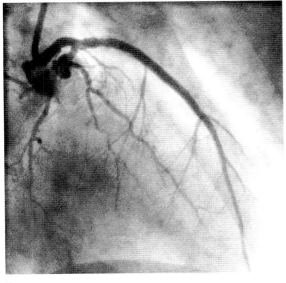

e

Figure 13.2 *continued*
c) After wire passage and inflation a 'flap-like' lesion is seen across LAD. d) Hazy appearance at site seen in c. e) After new stent deployed, resultant angiogram.

completely disrupt the clot but not to keep inflating to higher and higher pressures if bits of thrombus can still be seen attached within the stent. If there is a clear edge dissection then I would deploy an overlapping stent, as in this case, in order to cover it.

In any case of stent thrombosis it is important to document the degree of myocardial damage that has resulted from it. This should be done by both cardiac enzymes and echo assessment of LV function. Patients who had gone home and are transferred back into hospital are likely to have already sustained significant myocardial damage and need to be treated appropriately for this with ACE inhibitors. I would not routinely anticoagulate patients because they had had a stent thrombosis.

14
Restenosis

Restenosis represents a major challenge to the interventional community. We cause it, and even with the best results ever published the angiographic restenosis rate for stented vessels is still at least 10%! This chapter inevitably focuses on mechanisms for treating restenotic lesions, although perhaps it is more appropriate for the long term that we dedicate our resources towards understanding why some patients are susceptible to intimal proliferation, so that we may develop prophylactic strategies to prevent it.

Current treatment options are diverse and each interventionist has their own bias. Without doubt, further high quality randomized studies are required to help provide unequivocal guidance as to the correct therapy for this difficult patient group.

We invited **Patrick Serruys** and co-workers **Manel Sabaté** and **Jurgen MR Ligthart** to discuss the options for the management of restenosis, including the role of brachytherapy.

Case 1. Restenosis

55-year-old man. Ex-smoker; high cholesterol. Inferior MI 1997 treated with streptokinase. Recurrent angina since then with abnormal ETT.

Catheter findings: Good LV; single-vessel disease in dominant RCA with proximal occlusion.

Procedure: JR4 8F; 0.014″ high torque floppy wire. Extensive area dilated with 2.5 mm monorail balloon. Magic Wallstent® (48 mm) then deployed from proximal to mid-vessel and more distal lesion stented with Cordis CrossFlex® 3.0 mm × 25 mm.
Represented with limiting angina 5 months later when angiogram showed diffuse restenosis within the stents.
Procedure: JR4 8F; 0.014″ high torque floppy wire. Whole stented area dilated with 3.5 mm Chubby™ balloon to 16 atm.

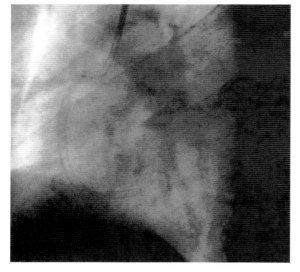

a

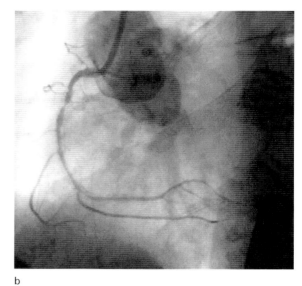

b

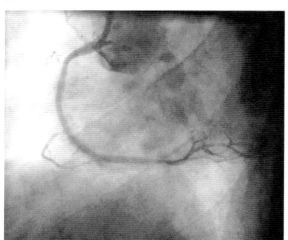

c

Figure 14.1
RCA angiogram. a) Acquisition of image, without contrast, to visualize Wallstent® in RCA. b) Diffuse in-stent restenosis with tight proximal segment. c) Result after extensive balloon dilatation.

Case 2. Restenosis

55-year-old man. Hypertension; hypercholesterol-aemia; ex-smoker; family history.
8/96 PTCA plus Cordis CrossFlex™ 3.5 mm × 15 mm to proximal LAD.
5/97 recurrent limiting angina.

Catheter findings: Significant stenosis in stent.

Procedure: JL4 8F guide; 0.014″ high torque floppy wire; 3.5 mm monorail balloon inflated within stent and above it. Then two ACS MULTI-LINK® stents as follows: (a) 3.5 mm × 35 mm to 12 atm deployed overlapping and extending distally from the original Cordis CrossFlex™; (b) 3.5 mm × 15 mm ACS MULTI-LINK® overlapping (a) proximally.

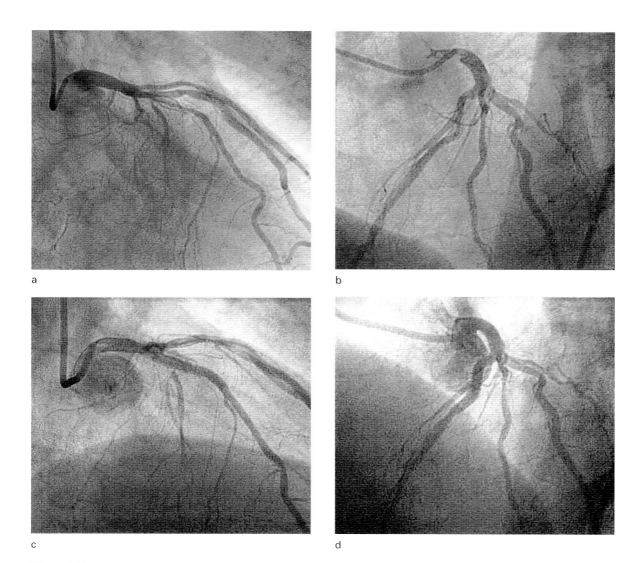

a

b

c

d

Figure 14.2
LCA angiogram. a) In-stent restenosis in LAD, PA projection. b) In-stent restenosis in LAD, LAO projection. c) After balloon dilatation and stent placed in stented territory, result in PA projection. d) Result in LAO projection.

Case 3. Restenosis

62-year-old man. Ex-smoker; hypertension. 7/96 PTCA plus stent to LAD. 5/97 recurrent limiting angina.

Catheter findings: Stenosis within stent.

Procedure: JL4 8F guide; 0.014″ high torque floppy wire; 3.5 mm monorail balloon inflated within stent and above it. The ACS MULTI-LINK® 3.5 mm × 25 mm overlapping whole of old stent.

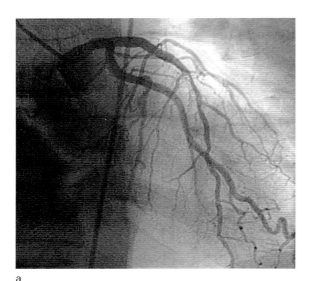

a

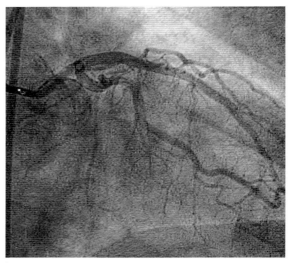

b

Figure 14.3
LCA angiogram. a) In-stent mid-LAD lesion. b) Dilated and restented.

Case 4. Restenosis

54-year-old man. High cholesterol; hypertension; ex-smoker. Acute anterior MI treated with streptokinase resulting in no Q wave. Stented, with recurrent symptoms at 6 months.

Catheter findings: Tight restenosis at site of stent with poor downstream run-off.

Procedure: LC4 8F, 0.014" high torque floppy wire; 3.0 mm monorail balloon at high pressure, 18 atm, with excellent angiographic result.

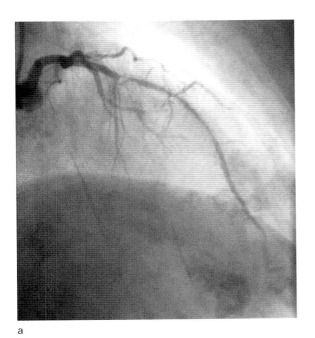

a

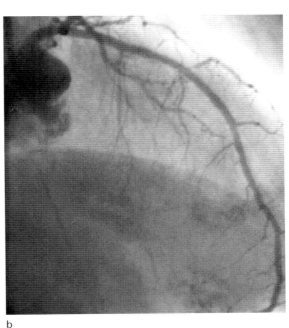

b

Figure 14.4
LCA angiogram. a) Mid-LAD lesion within stent at 6 months. b) Result after in-stent redilatation with 3.0 mm balloon at high pressure.

Case 5. Restenosis

76-year-old man. Ex-smoker. CABG surgery 1992 (vein grafts to LAD and RCA). Presented in 1996 with angina: underwent PTCA plus Medtronic Wiktor® 3.5 mm × 15 mm to AV circumflex. Presents again 9 months later with unstable angina.

Catheter findings: LV function poor with extensive

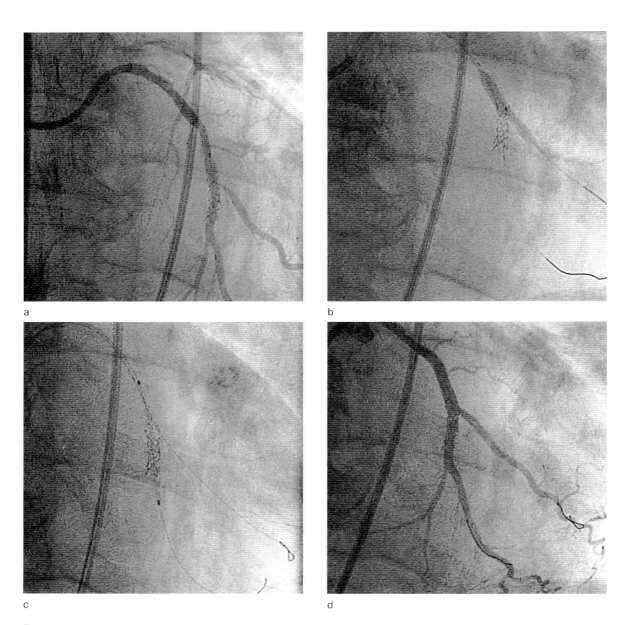

Figure 14.5
LCA angiogram. a) Selective circumflex injection: OM tight proximal stenosis. b) Guidewire to each limb and balloon to origin of OM, stent to Cx/OM. c) Stent through Cx/OM stent, into distal OM. d) Final result of true Y stent.

inferoapical hypokinesis; LAD occluded after first diagonal; in-stent stenosis involving origin of OM; severe proximal RCA disease; both vein grafts patent with good run off.

Procedure: Amplatz left 8F guide; 0.014" high torque floppy wire to AVCx and OM. IVUS confirmed very tight stenosis at OM origin and significant stenosis within body of Medtronic Wiktor®. Both AVCx and OM origin pre-dilated with 3.0 mm monorail balloon. Then 3.0 mm × 15 mm ACS MULTI-LINK® into OM1 from AVCx and 4.0 mm × 15 mm ACS MULTI-LINK® in AVCx across origin of OM (as a true 'Y' stent). Further 3.5 mm × 15 mm ACS MULTI-LINK® overlapping distal end of Cx stent.

Comments of Patrick Serruys, Manel Sabaté and Jurgen MR Ligthart:

This chapter addresses the controversial topic of the treatment of in-stent restenosis. Although restenosis is less frequent than after balloon angioplasty, the rate after stent implantation involves 15–20% in the best selected cases.[1,2] The mechanism of in-stent restenosis is basically neointimal proliferation, since the recoil and late vessel constriction is prevented by the mechanical properties of the stent.

The treatment of this complication involves various techniques, including balloon angioplasty in-stent, stent implantation in-stent, debulking techniques and more recently intracoronary radiation therapy. This variety of approaches illustrates that the problem is far from being solved. In the cases selected, the operators chose either treatment with balloon angioplasty or stent implantation within the restenosed stent, showing satisfactory angiographic results. However, the long-term follow-up of these patients is not presented. In fact, the recurrence rate appears to increase with the number of re-interventions performed on the lesion.

Debulking techniques appear to provide additional value to balloon angioplasty for the treatment of in-stent restenosis. For example, when compared to balloon angioplasty alone, laser debulking followed by balloon angioplasty demonstrated a greater lumen gain, more intimal

hyperplasia ablation/extrusion, larger lumen cross-sectional area and a tendency for less frequent need for subsequent target vessel revascularization.[3] In the same way, rotational atherectomy showed a lower clinical recurrence rate and a higher long-term angina-free survival when used concomitantly with balloon angioplasty as compared to balloon angioplasty alone.[4] Finally, treatment with atherectomy plus adjunctive balloon angioplasty resulted in higher acute gain and a trend towards a lower need for repeat target vessel revascularization.[5] A comparison of balloon angioplasty, laser and rotational atherectomy has recently been reported (oral presentation in the American Heart Association, 1998), showing better results by the use of adjunctive rotational atherectomy as compared to the other two approaches.

The recent introduction of intracoronary radiation in the therapeutic arsenal has provided the interventional cardiologist with a new approach to treat restenotic coronary lesions. The theoretical benefit of radiation in preventing neointimal proliferation resides in its ability to kill the more rapidly dividing smooth muscle cells. To date, two randomized placebo-controlled trials have been carried out to evaluate the efficacy of gamma-radiation in patients with in-stent restenosis.[6,7] Teirstein et al.[6] randomized 55 patients to receive a 0.030" ribbon containing ^{192}Ir sealed sources or a ribbon containing placebo seeds (Best Industries, Springfield, VA). Thirty-five patients were treated with in-stent restenosis. The dosimetry was calculated from the intravascular ultrasound measurement in a range of 8–30 Gray to the internal elastic membrane. The placebo group showed a restenosis rate of 70% as compared to 14% in the irradiated group ($p = 0.0006$). This beneficial effect was sustained at 2-year follow-up. Waksman et al.[7] evaluated 130 patients who had developed in-stent restenosis up to 47 mm long in the Washington Radiation for In-stent Restenosis Trial (WRIST). These patients were randomized to radiation using a ^{192}Ir ribbon versus a non-radioactive ribbon delivered into a non-centred closed-end lumen catheter (Medtronic, San Diego, CA). The prescribed dose was 15 Gray to a distance of 2 mm from the centre of the source for a vessel size of 3.0–4.0 mm and to a distance of 2.4 mm from the centre of the source for vessel diameter of 4.0–5.0 mm. At 6-month follow-up, the

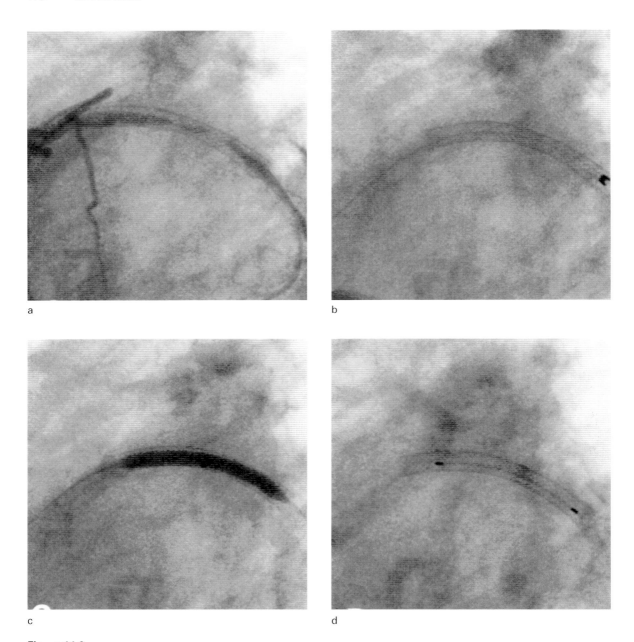

Figure 14.6
LCA angiogram. a) In-stent restenosis with a Wallstent™. b) Laser catheter in distal stent. c) Post-laser dilatation. d) 'Hot-wire' in stent, markers at each end of 'hot' segment.

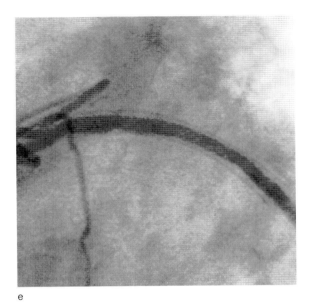

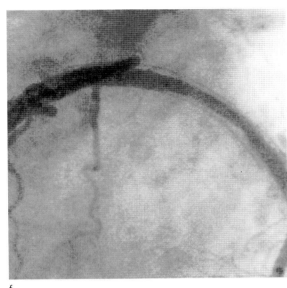

e

f

Figure 14.6 *continued*
e) Final angiogram. f) Six-month follow-up angiogram.

irradiated group showed a reduction of 67% in the restenosis rate, 79% reduction in total lesion revascularization requirement and 63% reduction in major adverse cardiac events.

Although the use of beta radiation is easier to implement in the catheterization laboratory, it presents the potential drawback of the steep dose fall-off, which might lead to heterogeneity of the prescribed dose to the vessel wall and potentially less impressive results. In our experience, 18 consecutive patients with recurrent in-stent restenosis have been treated by the use of the Beta-Cath System™ (Novoste Corp. Norcross, GA). Ten patients were pre-treated with laser debulking followed by adjunctive balloon angioplasty and eight pre-treated with balloon angioplasty alone. To date 14 patients have returned for 6-month angiographic follow-up. Seven patients (50%) presented in-stent restenosis (> 50% diameter stenosis), resulting in target vessel revascularization in six of them. An example of a patient treated with laser, followed by beta-radiation is depicted in Figs 14.6a–e. The follow-up angiogram is depicted in Fig. 14.6f.

A more provocative approach would be the implantation of a radioactive stent within the restenosed stent. This approach would add the beneficial effect of the stent in preventing recoil of the neointimal hyperplasia and the theoretical effect of the radiation in preventing tissue proliferation.

In conclusion, treatment of in-stent restenosis remains a challenge for the interventional cardiologist. Ideally, the combination of balloon angioplasty, debulking techniques and intracoronary radiation would present an additive effect resulting in an improvement of the recurrence of this complication. Further randomized trials should address the effectiveness of this combined approach in the treatment of in-stent restenosis.

Editors' note

A further therapeutic option for in-stent restenosis is the cutting balloon (IVT Europe). Preliminary data suggest that the initial angiographic result obtained is superior to that of conventional POBA[8] and furthermore that angiographic restenosis may be significantly lower with the device.[9,10] Various theoretical mechanisms of benefit are suggested, including the hypothesis that the cutting balloon reduces vessel wall trauma and thereby attenuates the local balloon-induced vascular inflammatory response.[11]

References

1. Fischman DL, Leon MB, Baim DS, et al. A randomized comparison of coronary-stent placement in the treatment of coronary artery disease. Stent Restenosis Study Investigators. N Engl J Med 1994;331:496–501.
2. Serruys PW, de Jaegere P, Kiemeneij F, et al. A comparison of balloon expandable-stent implantation with balloon angioplasty in patients with coronary artery disease. N Engl J Med 1994;331:489–495.
3. Mehran R, Mintz GS, Satler LF, et al. Treatment of in-stent restenosis with excimer laser coronary angioplasty. Circulation 1997:96:2183–2189.
4. Lee SG, Lee CW, Cheong SS, et al. Immediate and long-term outcomes of rotational atherectomy versus balloon angioplasty alone for treatment of diffuse in-stent restenosis. Am J Cardiol 1998;15:140–143.
5. Dauerman HL, Baim DS, Cutlip DE, et al. Mechanical debulking versus balloon angioplasty for the treatment of diffuse in-stent restenosis. Am J Cardiol 1998;82:277–284.
6. Teirstein PS, Massulo V, Shirish J, et al. Catheter-based radiotherapy to inhibit restenosis after coronary stenting. N Engl J Med 1997;336:1697–1703.
7. Waksman R, White LR, Chan RC, et al. Intracoronary radiation therapy for patients with in-stent restenosis: 6 month follow up of a randomized clinical study. Circulation 1998;98 (Suppl):I-651 (abstract).
8. Chevalier B, Royer T, Guyon P et al. Treatment of in-stent restenosis: results of a randomised study between balloon and cutting balloon. TCT 1998, poster 192.
9. Suzuki T. The usefulness of cutting balloon angioplasty for in-stent restenosis: comparison with POBA. TCT 1998; oral presentation.
10. Nakamura M, Suzuki T, Matsubara T, et al. Results of cutting balloon angioplasty for stent restenosis. Japanese multicentre registry. J Am Coll Cardiol 1998;31(Suppl A):235A.
11. Inoue T, Sakai Y, Hoshi, et al. Lower expression of neutrophil adhesion molecule indicates less vessel wall injury and might explain lower restenosis rate after cutting balloon angioplasty. Circulation 1998;97:2511–2518.

15
Local drug delivery from coated stents

The issue of prevention and treatment of restenosis, whether it occurs following balloon angioplasty, stent insertion, or other therapeutic endeavour, is the goal of the scientist involved in the management of coronary artery disease. The invaluable legacy of Andreas Gruntzig and John Simpson in the pioneering work that initiated the practice of coronary angioplasty, and spawned all of the interventional techniques and practices of today, is only held back by the remaining major issue of restenosis. This remaining barrier leads to negative impact on patients and health economics.

The scientific community are expending enormous energy on the issue of overcoming restenosis; we have asked renowned workers in the area to combine to give their views on where the science currently stands, and where it will lead.

We invited Drs **Anthony H Gershlick**, **Julia Baron**, **Johanna Armstrong**, **Neil Swanson**, **Christopher MH Newman** and **Cathy Holt** to predict the value of stent coatings:

Coronary stenting is associated with lower rates of restenosis than balloon angioplasty.[1,2] Restenosis following angioplasty is a combination of recoil, negative remodelling and intimal hyperplasia which involves a combination of proliferative smooth muscle cells and extracellular matrix. Stents address the first two components of restenosis but do not influence the development of intimal tissue, which IVUS studies have shown to occur to a greater extent within stents than after angioplasty. The development of intimal smooth muscle cell hyperplasia is thus the cause of the 10% and 15% incidence of in-stent restenosis.

Stent use has grown exponentially. Currently there are 1,200,000 percutaneous interventions undertaken annually world-wide. An average stent use of 70% means that up to 100,000 interventions are required to treat in-stent restenosis. In some patients the intimal smooth muscle cell proliferation has a greater clinical impact. Either it is exaggerated (as in diabetics who suffer restenosis rates of up to 45%[3]) or it may have proportionally more impact, as in patients with small reference diameters. Treating in-stent intimal hyperplasia with repeat balloon angioplasty can be very difficult, especially if the hyperplasia is diffusely distributed, with reported re-restenosis rates of >50%.

The nature of restenosis following stenting makes treating it, or perhaps more importantly preventing its initial occurrence, intellectually and scientifically challenging. Current effective therapies consist essentially of radiation treatment, which is not without its complications (potential in-stent thrombosis, delayed endothelial healing, edge effects, and adverse long term positive vessel remodelling). Brachytherapy as currently applied is essentially secondary prevention. The difference between stenting and surgery in the ARTS trial[4] (14% greater repeat revascularization rates in the stent group) was due to intimal hyperplasia (causing in-stent restenosis) and was a factor in reducing the cost effectiveness of stenting.

It is clear that a cheap and effective method of effecting primary prevention is required. Delivering stents that elute drugs which can beneficially influence the pathobiology of in-stent intimal hyperplasia is thus an attractive concept.

Stent thrombosis is now rare but still occurs and carries with it a significant adverse morbidity. Routinely administered and effective oral antiplatelet therapy is expensive and not without side-effects. Thus a second goal for stent-based drug delivery might be the development of a stent that is truly non-thrombogenic, and one that can be deployed under any clinical circumstances (small calibre vessel, patient presenting with acute coronary syndrome), without the need to systemically administer powerful and expensive intravenous anti-platelet agents.

Minimal requirements for successful stent-based local drug delivery

Lessons from studies of balloon-based local drug delivery suggest that, for the stent based concept to be successful the following criteria need to be met:

- The drug should retain maximal biological efficacy when loaded
- Sufficient drug should be carried on the stent to achieve high local tissue concentrations
- Active drug should be bio-available to the target cell rather than the vessel wall layer (e.g. media versus adventitia)
- The agent should elute from the stent at a rate that allows it to be available over the time course of the pathological response (for up to 2 weeks in the case of smooth muscle cell migration and proliferation)
- Active agent cannot be irreversibly bound to the struts since it will be required in those areas of the vessel wall not covered by stent strut (~85%)
- Ideally the drug used should have minimal effects on other cell types (such as endothelial cells)
- Activity of the agent and quantity of the drug retained on the stent should not be influenced by any necessary processes such as sterilization, shipping times, storage or intra-arterial blood flow
- Modifications of the stent to enable drug delivery should not adversely influence the performance of the stent, as in excluding side-branch access or its ability to track, nor should the process of drug attachment itself exaggerate any cellular reaction to the stent
- Proof of principle, effectiveness and safety should be established in in-vitro and animal work before pilot clinical studies are undertaken

Current status of local delivery of drug with stents

Enabling stents to deliver agents

The choices are to bind the agent to the bare metal or to incorporate the drug into a polymer or coating. Initial work using a stent as a local drug-delivery device utilized the Carmeda AB principle to avidly bind heparin to the polymer-coated stent. While work in a pig model demonstrated efficacy, the clinical trial (BENESTENT II) was limited by the absence of a control group. Even taking account of this the principle of binding the drug so avidly to the stent would suggest that the intrastrut spaces would not be treated. Polymers that allow the drug to elute off the stent into the surrounding tissue may be a better option. Air-drying drugs onto bare metal is an alternative option that is currently being considered.

Extensive research has been undertaken into assessing the feasibility and applicability of using different polymer coatings as a way of delivering drugs with stents (Fig. 15.1). Drug elution from polymer-coated stents is, theoretically, an ideal system, as it combines drug carriage with local delivery of a high concentration of agents and sustained release. The polymer acts as a drug reservoir and the subsequent drug delivery may be by simple diffusion, by degradation of the polymer, or by cleavage of drug from the polymer.[5] Variations in polymer characteristics, for example adjusting pore size, can be made to accommodate different drug molecular weights and different elution rates. Indeed, drug-eluting polymer stents have been used in experimental animal studies with promising results, but the first principle of there needing to be no adverse effects as a result of the modifications for delivering the drug needs to apply. Thus, first and foremost polymer coatings need to be biologically neutral.

Polymer coatings

Several polymers previously used in medicine have been evaluated for their suitability as stent coatings. Van der Giesson et al.[6] investigated eight different polymers with respect to their

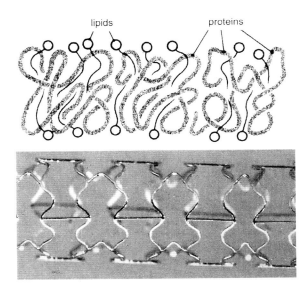

Figure 15.1
The structure of a typical polymer. The stent shown is polymer coated and has no effect on the stent performance

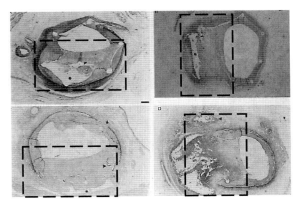

Figure 15.2
Marked inflammatory changes (in boxes) with some polymers. In this study by van der Giessen et al.[6] half the stent was coated with polymer and the other half acted as control. The inflammatory response is clearly seen

biocompatibility. A severe inflammatory response was reported after deployment of all of these stents in porcine coronary arteries (Fig. 15.2). Poly(organo)phosphazene polymers were also shown to initiate a foreign body reaction in porcine arteries.[7] Poly-L-lactic acid (PLLA) has also been used to coat stents, and these experiments demonstrated an inflammatory reaction with low molecular weight PLLA, but not with high molecular weight PLLA.[8] Polymers incorporating naturally occurring lipids, for instance phosphorylcholine (PC) (Fig. 15.3), have also been used as a stent coating by Cumberland and others.[9] PC-containing polymers have the benefit of reducing platelet activation and adhesion and may also be used as drug-delivery platforms. PC does not invoke a significant inflammatory response[10] and does not increase the neointimal response to stenting in the pig model.[11] Other bioneutral polymers include the chlorohydrocarbon used to coat the Cook stent. This polymer has been extensively tested in our laboratory and provides reproducible adsorption and elution profiles with a number of potentially beneficial agents including c7E3-Fab,[12] Activated Protein C,[13] and vascular endothelial growth factor (VEGF).[14]

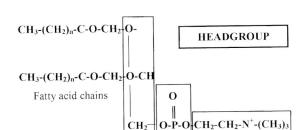

Figure 15.3
The construct of phosphorylcholine, a non-inflammatory polymer derived from the red blood cell membrane

Being able to adapt polymer structure means that there is the potential to enable drugs with different molecular size to be delivered over variable elution periods. Thus the stent-device may be tailored to the requirements of the agent being delivered or the process being targeted.

Methods of drug loading and elution

The type of drug binding and its elution profile are important considerations when delivering drugs from stents. For some agents a 'one hit' strategy may be considered appropriate (e.g. paclitaxel or rapamycin) whereas slower release may be more appropriate for other drugs such as heparin. Polymers may even be designed to allow a combination and perhaps in the future may be loaded with more than one agent.

Drug *absorption* refers to the incorporation of a drug into a matrix, which is then applied to the stent surface as a coating. The drug and polymer are blended together, and drug release can be modified by altering the proportion of hydrophilic polymers, the degree of cross-linking and the type of plasticizer used.[15] The potential problems with such methods include denaturation of the agent during the process of blending. Advantages include the ability to load greater quantities of drug and having some control over the elution characteristics.

Drug *adsorption* refers to the method of layering a drug onto the polymer coating of a stent. In both absorption and adsorption, the drug is attached to the polymer by either covalent or non-covalent bonds. A positively charged polymer can be used to ionically bind a negatively charged drug. A more stable attachment of the drug to the polymer is achieved through covalent bonding. Rather than simple passive release, the drug may be removed through interaction of the drug with its target molecule. In addition to ionic and covalent interactions, the polymer matrix may passively take up the drug into spaces between the polymer molecules. Passive adsorption through a process not dissimilar to the ELISA technique may be a benign and thus valuable way of loading stents. The disadvantage is that the quantity that can be passively loaded will be limited and variable (Fig. 15.4).

The way in which a drug is incorporated into a polymer stent coating determines the way in which it is released. Random release describes

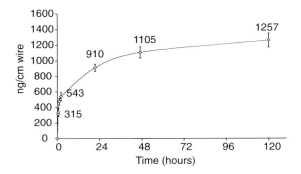

Figure 15.4
2 mg/ml, 25°C, no buffer exchange. Uptake of drug (c7E3-Fab) into a polymer-coated stent through passive adsorption is dose and time related, but eventually a plateau is reached

diffusion of the drug from the polymer matrix and is dependent on the thickness of the coating and the amount of drug incorporated.[16] Controlled drug release can also be achieved if the matrix is a biodegradable polymer.[8] The rate of polymer degradation determines the rate of drug release. Most ongoing work involves the active incorporation into proprietary polymers that allow sustained, controlled, and predictable release of drug from the stent into the vessel wall. Depth of release remains an under-investigated problem. Even in stented arteries plaque distribution may still be eccentric. Therefore, the deep medial layers may be differentially treated.

Experience with polymer coated stents

Basic science

Various molecules of differing characteristics have been successfully loaded onto polymer coated stents via passive uptake (Table 15.1). Generally, the molecule to be investigated may be detected using techniques such as fluoroscopy, radioactivity or HPLC analysis. A molecule may be naturally fluorescent (such as dipyridamole) or may be tagged with a fluorescent label and then localized by ultraviolet

Table 15.1. Agents delivered from coated stents

Drug	Biological action	Size (MW)	Solubility	Method of detection
Dipyridamole	Inhibitor of platelet aggregation Vasodilator Reduces smooth muscle cell proliferation.	504	Hydrophobic	Fluorescence microscopy
Angiopeptin	Reduces neointima formation in animal models Reduced clinical events in a human trial	1067	Hydrophilic	Labelled with radio-isotopic iodine (^{125}I)
ReoPro® (c7E3 Fab)	Potent anti-platelet agent Inhibits smooth muscle cell migration Reduces incidence of coronary events post-PTCA	47615	Hydrophilic	Immunohistochemical detection
Dexamethasone	Anti-inflammatory Inhibits neointima formation in animal models	393	Hydrophobic	Labelled with radio-isotopic hydrogen (^{3}H)

microscopy and quantified by fluorimetry. Some molecules may be radiolabelled (e.g. angiopeptin) and subsequently localized by autoradiography and quantified by counting of radioactivity. In order to determine that it is not simply a cleaved tag that is being detected, techniques such as HPLC analysis may be performed to determine the intactness of the delivered agent.

Estimation of loading and elution characteristics in vitro may be best assessed by radio-labelling techniques. Thus the uptake and loss of VEGF for example can be easily quantitated in an in-vitro rig with bovine serum albumin or blood as the medium. Such studies show that many drugs taken up passively into a polymer have a bi-exponential loss (Fig. 15.5), the steep part of any such curve being more likely to be due to loss into the circulation rather than into the tissue.

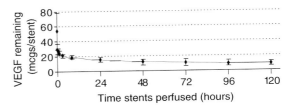

Figure 15.5
Bi-exponential loss of vascular endothelial growth factor from a polymer-coated stent

Which agents to load

There are currently a number of agents being tested at different stages from bench studies to early clinical trials. Most agents being evaluated are known to affect smooth muscle proliferation, migration, or both. Some, such as c7E3-Fab (abciximab) have other properties. This agent has shown powerful antiplatelet activity. It is currently used clinically to treat arterial thrombus, and is administered either prophylactically

or after thrombus has formed, for example as occurs with stent thrombosis. There are good data to suggest that the administration of abciximab will reduce the potentially adverse prognostic enzyme 'bumps' that indicate micro-infarction following routine stenting, and its use will favourably influence PCI in diabetics. It makes a good candidate for local drug delivery, since its systemic use adds significantly to the cost of the procedure, and systemic bleeding, especially from the arterial puncture site, can and does occur when it is given intravenously.

The efficacy of stent-delivered glycoprotein IIb/IIIa receptor blockers on in-vitro platelet function and in-vivo stent thrombosis has been tested. AZ1 is an inhibitor of the platelet glyco-protein IIb/IIIa receptor[17] and is one that has been tested to establish the in-vivo benefit of drug eluting stents. The aim was to determine whether

AZ1-loaded stents beneficially altered the interaction between the stent, the damaged vessel
wall, and the circulating blood. The antibody was
passively adsorbed onto cellulose polymer-
coated stents, and these were implanted in
balloon-damaged flow-reduced arteries. Control
stents (either base polymer alone or a stent
loaded with irrelevant antibody adsorbed in a
similar manner) were implanted in the opposite
rabbit iliac artery. The biological effect was
demonstrated with a significant improvement in
the patency rate at both 2 hours and 28 days (AZ1
adsorbed stents patency rate 100% versus 40%, *p*
= 0.015).[18] The AZ1 was adsorbed passively onto
the stent by a simple dipping technique, and its
elution, an important prerequisite for influencing
the stent interstitial spaces, had been shown in
vitro to follow a reproducible gradual bi-exponential pattern. This demonstration of 'proof of
principle' has importantly fulfilled all the criteria
listed above as being required for successful
stent-based drug delivery.

Further work with c7E3-Fab, the human equivalent of AZ1, showed that the adsorption and
elution followed a similar pattern to that of AZ1,
with 52% of the original amount adsorbed still
being present after 12 days of continual perfusion[12] (Fig. 15.6). Baron et al has shown that in
the doses that might be delivered after loading
onto a stent, it has profound anti-platelet effects.[19]

How may c7E3-Fab loaded stents be of value?
Currently abciximab is used in Europe in about
30% of patients being stented. Most centres use
it reactively when stent deployment cannot be
made ideal or there is clear evidence of thrombus formation. Such decisions are driven by cost
issues, despite the evidence of potential benefit
from studies such as EPISTENT.[20] Beneficial
outcome is likely to be due to the reduction in
microembolic small-vessel occlusions. Whether
enzyme rises can be reduced by stents being
loaded with such powerful glycoprotein IIb/IIIa
receptor blockers in humans needs to be tested
in appropriately designed clinical trials.

Additionally, ab7E3-Fab is worth considering
as an agent for local delivery since it is thought
to have effects other than those on platelets. For
example, it affects integrins on white blood cells
and on smooth muscle cells. The integrin family
consists of molecules composed of a series of α
and β subunits. When combined, these form
receptors that mediate a wide variety of cell

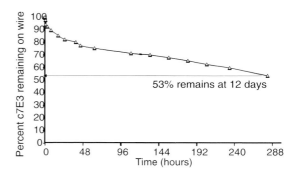

Figure 15.6
*20 min adsorption, 2.0 ml, coating buffer, room temp. Loss
of c7E3-Fab from a polymer-coated stent. Drug elutes over
a period of more than 2 weeks, which is the ideal time for
inhibiting smooth muscle cell activity if inhibition of the
biological process requires constant exposure to the
inhibitory agent*

functions via specific ligands. One of the main
integrins on smooth muscle cells responsible for
mediating their migration is the $\alpha_v\beta_3$ integrin.
This shares a β_3 subunit with the glycoprotein
IIb/IIIa integrin present on platelets. It has been
shown that 7E3, which inhibits the α_{IIb}/β_3 on
platelets does indeed cross-react with the
smooth muscle cell integrin through the shared
β_3. If drugs such as abciximab can block platelet
glycoprotein IIb/IIIa receptors they may influence
the β_3 receptor on the smooth muscle cells to
beneficially influence restenosis. Studies on the
effects of the monoclonal antibody on human
vascular smooth muscle cell function in vitro
have shown similar inhibition of cell adhesion
and migration to that seen with other anti-$\alpha_v\beta_3$
antibodies.[21] If such techniques can be repro-
duced in vivo then a truly non-thrombogenic,
non-restenosing stent may be a possibility.
Abciximab-loaded stents are unaffected by sterilization fulfilling another of the criteria for
successful stent based drug delivery.

A clinical trial of c7E3-Fab-eluting stents in
patients with stents placed in small vessels (high

risk for thrombosis and restenosis) is planned (the ReoPro® in Small Vessels [RESOLVE] trial). It is likely that this study will use the PC-coated biocompatible stent which has a CE mark for drug loading.

Other agents tested include activated protein C, a potent antithrombotic,[22] and VEGF. Evidence suggests that endothelial damage is in part responsible for thrombosis/restenosis. Endothelial recovery takes up to 2 weeks and during this time the PCI site is vulnerable to complications, including thrombosis and intimal hyperplasia leading to the development of restenosis. VEGF is an endothelium specific mitogen. Previous animal studies have examined the effects of VEGF when given as a local infusion using a delivery balloon to the PCI site. These studies suggested that VEGF would promote endothelial regrowth at the site and so might reduce stent complications, particularly intimal hyperplasia.[23] This is thought to be due to a more rapid 'passivation' of the stent as endothelial cells grow over it. A further study using the same techniques showed that, not only was the endothelial integrity restored, but the regenerated endothelium was functional, at least for restoring vasomotor responsiveness and thromboresistance.[24] The potential to deliver VEGF with stents has been evaluated using polymer-coated stents. Maximum adsorption of 53.8 ± 24 μg VEGF/stent was shown after 48 hours of passive soaking in a 2-mg/ml solution of VEGF. Initial rapid release of VEGF was seen, whereas late VEGF release from stents was much slower.[25] These data showed that polymer-coated stents could deliver VEGF locally and in a sustained fashion. Thus VEGF delivered from a polymer-coated stent might potentially encourage rapid re-endothelialization. The use of such stents may be of critical value following brachytherapy,[26] where the longer term effects of the prolonged de-endothelialization are unknown. Adverse effects on stent thrombosis have been significant enough to necessitate prolonging the administration of anti-platelet therapy from 14 days for routine stenting to 90 days for stenting in the setting of brachytherapy. Some authors are suggesting that anti-platelet therapy should be 'forever' or until the patient suffers a side-effect from the anti-platelet agent.

For each agent tested it has been possible to load the stents in a reliable manner, and the elution profile is predictable.

Ex-vivo model of local drug delivery from phosphorylcholine-coated stents

The work undertaken on PC-coated stents in Sheffield demonstrates the steps that need to be undertaken to provide the link between in vitro work and clinical trials. In the Sheffield laboratory, PC-coated stents have been loaded with various drugs and have been deployed into segments of human or porcine vascular tissue using conventional methods. The stented vessels are subsequently cannulated at both ends and secured into a pulsatile flow circuit.[27] The flow circuit is perfused via a pump for various time intervals, and drug release into the circulating fluid is assessed in addition to localization of drug delivery into the vascular tissue (Figs 15.7 and 15.8).

Local drug delivery from phosphorylcholine-coated stents in vivo: the pig stent model

The pig model is a good one for testing drug eluting stents in vivo, although for some agents such as abciximab non-primate models are required. In the pig model carotid or coronary arteries can be used. In Sheffield, the studies involve cut-down on the carotid artery using standard procedures. Drug-loaded stents have also been implanted into pig coronary arteries. Animals may be killed at various time intervals after stent implantation and localization and quantification of delivered drug determined[28] (Fig. 15.9).

Clinical trials

The need to prevent restenosis rather than to treat it once it has occurred, together with the promising in-vitro and animal data, has led to an explosion of interest in stent-based drug delivery. Issues such as cost saving and reduced side-effects together with the early clinical studies have led to the initiation of a number of clinical trials.

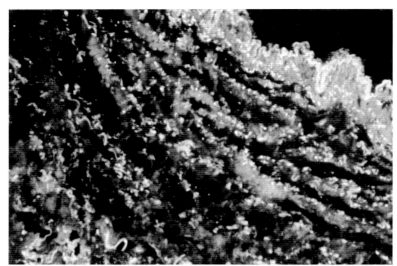

a

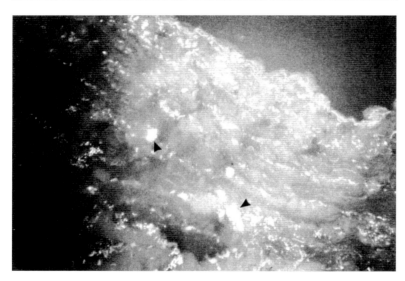

b

Figure 15.7
Location of dipyridamole delivered into human saphenous vein ex vivo and detected by fluorescence microscopy. Dipyridamole is naturally autofluorescent and may be detected by ultraviolet microscopy. (a) Control saphenous vein showing autofluorescence of elastic material within the vessel wall. (b) Central or stented segment of saphenous vein showing areas of fluorescent dipyridamole within the media 24 hours after stent deployment (arrows). Magnification × 320

Grube et al. have recently presented clinical findings on 32 patients treated with either control stents or paclitaxel-eluting stents; the restenosis rates were respectively 54% and 0%.[29] Because of the patient numbers, this study has the value of only demonstrating the potential of this combination and the need for a proper clinical trial, but the data are nevertheless intriguing.

There are two further studies underway or about to start that address the issue of in-stent restenosis using agents that have been shown in vitro, ex vivo and in animal studies to influence smooth muscle cell activity.

Paclitaxel has clinical use in ovarian cancer. It was discovered as part of a National Cancer Institute programme in which thousands of plants were screened for anti-cancer activity. In 1963 an extract from the bark of the Pacific yew (*Taxus brevifolia*), a relatively rare plant, was found to have cytotoxic activity against many tumours. It

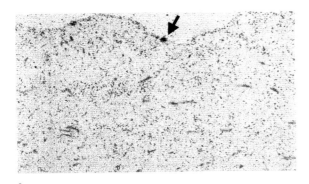

a

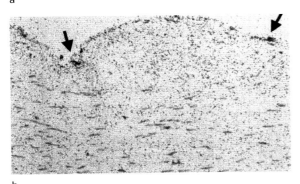

b

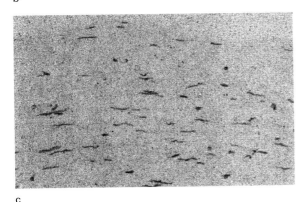

c

Figure 15.8
Location of [125I]angiopeptin delivered to human saphenous vein ex vivo. After 1 hour, dense areas of black silver grains representing [125I]angiopeptin can be seen in both proximal and central regions of the vein (a and b, arrowheads). No [125I]angiopeptin can be seen in the distal region (c). Magnification × 200

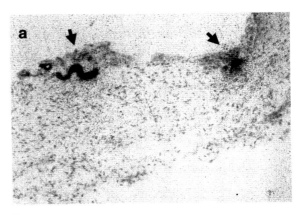

a

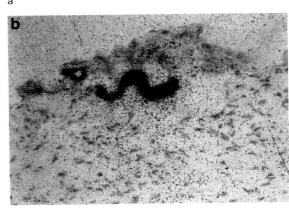

b

Figure 15.9
Location of [125I]angiopeptin delivered to porcine coronary arteries in vivo. (a,b) Microautoradiographs show the presence of [125I]angiopeptin (arrowheads) along the luminal surface, and extending a short distance into the media of the vessel directly surrounding the stent at 7 days (b (magnification × 320) = high power of a (magnification × 64)). [125I]Angiopeptin was seen at intermittent points along the intima, probably corresponding to the location of the stent struts prior to their removal

has specific properties against microtubules, promoting polymerization of tubulin. It inhibits the disassembly of microtubules, which thus become very stable and dysfunctional, so inhibiting cell division through inhibition of the mitotic spindle and cell death through its prevention of normal interphase functions.[30] Being a potent agent, with systemic side-effects, it is ideally suited to be considered for local, stent based delivery. As early as 1995 Sollott and others[31] had demonstrated inhibition of neointimal hyperplasia following angioplasty in the rat carotid artery model. We have now been able to coat stents with paclitaxel. In the pig coronary stent model the inhibitory effects on smooth muscle activity appear to be dose related with an inhibitory, but not necessarily linear, response (between 10 μg and 90 μg per stent). This, together with the dose-related inhibitory effects on post-traumatic endothelial cell regeneration, have led at this stage to the initiation of a European pilot safety study with the Cook V-Flex stent (the Evaluation of Taxol® Eluting Stent trial [ELUTES]). A further trial using the Boston Scientific stent and Taxol® is due to start in the Autumn of 2000.

A large European based trial of a drug called sirolimus has also started (the RAVEL study) following intriguing data from early clinical trials in South America. Sirolimus is a naturally occurring macrocyclic lactone. It has been used as an immunosupressive agent in renal and islet grafting and for bone marrow transplantation. It binds to a specific cytosolic protein (immunophilin) found in target cells. This complex then binds to a specific regulatory kinase called the 'mammalian target of rapamycin' (mTOR), inhibiting its activation, which in turn through inhibition of cell cycle progression suppresses cytokine-stimulated T-cell proliferation. However it has other effects, including inhibition of the translation of cdk4/cyclin d and cdk2/cyclin E complexes, that are perhaps of greater potential for inhibiting in-stent restenosis. Again the issues of local retention, safety and rate of re-endothelialization may be important. The doses of the agents used are minute compared to those administered systemically. Early results from the RAVEL study presented to the investigators are promising.

Summary and future directions

In-stent restenosis remains a major limitation to the long term success of coronary stenting. The ability to inhibit its formation via drug eluting stents is an attractive concept. Various polymers have been investigated as stent coatings capable of being loaded with therapeutic agents. Proof of the concept with various stents and a number of agents in vitro and in vivo have led to the initiation of early clinical trials. Candidate agents for inhibiting in-stent restenosis include not only traditional pharmacological agents, but also

gene therapy approaches.[32] One of the problems of such an approach is the delivery of genetic material in high amounts at the required site. Stent-based delivery may indeed provide the solution. However, further work aimed at elucidating the ideal therapeutic candidate is required before the promise of drug-eluting stents for the inhibition of in-stent restenosis may be delivered. Altering the drug, its concentration and the stent is relatively easy and cheap. Current stent user-friendliness appears to be unaffected.

Stent-based local drug delivery is the next important phase of stent development and it is likely that drug-eluting stents will become part of routine clinical practice.

References

1. Gershlick AH, Baron J. Dealing with in-stent restenosis. Heart 1998;79:319–323.
2. Serruys PW, de Jaegere P, Kiemeneij F, et al. for the Benestent Study Group. A comparison of balloon-expandable stent implantation with balloon angioplasty in patients with coronary disease. N Engl J Med 1994:331:489–495.
3. Van Belle E, Bauters C, Hubert E, et al. Restenosis rates in diabetic patients: a comparison of stenting and balloon angioplasty in native coronary vessels. Circulation 1997;96:1454–1460.
4. Serruys PW, Unger F, van Hout BA, et al. The ARTS study (Arterial Revascularization Therapies Study). Semin Intervent Cardiol 1999;4:209–219.
5. Eccleston D, Horrigan M, Ellis S. Rationale for local drug delivery. Semin Interven Cardiol 1996;8–16.
6. Van der Giessen WJ, Lincoff M, Schwartz R, et al. Marked inflammatory sequelae to implantation of biodegradable and non-biodegradable polymers in porcine coronary arteries. Circulation 1996;94:1690–1697.
7. De Scheeder I, Wilkzek K, Van Dorpe J, et al Local angiopeptin delivery using coated stents reduces neointimal proliferation in overstretched porcine coronary arteries. J Invasive Cardiol 1996;8:215–222.
8. Lincoff AM, Furst JG, Ellis SG, Tuch RJ, Topol EJ. Sustained local delivery of dexamethasone by a novel intravascular eluting stent to prevent restenosis in the porcine coronary injury model. J Am Coll Cardiol 1997;29:808–816.
9. Cumberland DC, Gunn J, Malik N, Holt CM. Biomimicry 1: PC. Semin Intervent Cardiol 1998;3:149–150.
10. Malik N, Gunn J, Shepherd L, et al. Phosphorylcholine-coated stents in porcine

coronary arteries: angiographic and morphometric assessment. Eur Heart J 1997;18:152(abstract).

11. Whelan DM, van der Giessen WJ, Krabbendam SC, van Vliet EA, et al. Biocompatibility of phosphorylcholine coated stents in normal porcine coronary arteries. Heart 2000;83:338–345.

12. Baron JH, Aggrawal R, de Bono DP, Gershlick AH. Adsorption and elution of c7E3 Fab from polymer coated stents in-vitro. ESC 1997 (abstract).

13. Foo RS, Hogrefe K, Baron JH, de Bono DP, Gershlick AH. Activated protein C to prevent thrombosis in percutaneous coronary intervention. Clin Sci 1999;96(Suppl 40):4P(abstract).

14. Swanson N, Hogrefe K, Baron J, et al. VEGF-eluting stents to reduce stent complications—pharmacokinetics of adsorption and elution. 6th International LDD&R Local Drug delivery meeting and cardiovascular course on radiation and molecular strategies 28/1/2000 (abstract).

15. Shargul L, Yu ABC. Applied Biopharmaceutics and Pharmacokinetics, 3rd Edn. Prentice Hall International, 1993.

16. Lambert T, Dev V, Rechavia E, Forrester J, et al. Localised arterial wall drug delivery from a polymer-coated removable metallic stent. Kinetics, distribution and bioactivity of forskolin. Circulation 1994;90:1003–1011.

17. Azrin MA, Ling FS, Chen Q, et al. Preparation, characterization, and evaluation of a monoclonal antibody against the rabbit platelet glycoprotein IIb/IIIa in an experimental angioplasty model. Circ Res 1994;75:268–277.

18. Aggarwal RK, Ireland DC, Azrin MA, et al. Antithrombotic potential of polymer-coated stents eluting platelet glycoprotein IIb/IIIa receptor antibody. Circulation. 1996;94:3311–3317.

19. Baron JH, de Bono DP, Gershlick AH. Adsorption of c7E3 Fab onto polymer-coated Cook GR II stents: Reopro eluting stents inhibit platelet deposition in vitro. Heart 1998;55:183(abstract).

20. Lincoff AM. Potent complementary clinical benefit of abciximab and stenting during percutaneous coronary revascularisation in patients with diabetes mellitus. Results of the EPISTENT study. Am Heart J 2000;139:S46–52(Review).

21. Baron JH, Aggrawal R, de Bono DP, Gershlick AH. c7E3 Fab inhibits adhesion of smooth muscle cells to vitronectin: a possible way of inhibiting in-stent restenosis. ESC 1997 (abstract).

22. Foo RS, Gershlick AH, Hogrefe K, et al. Inhibition of platelet thrombosis using an activated protein C-loaded stent: in vitro and in vivo results. Thromb Haemost 2000;83:496–502.

23. Van Belle E, Tio FO, Chen D, et al. Passivation of metallic stents after arterial gene transfer of phVEGF165 inhibits thrombus formation and intimal thickening. J Am Coll Cardiol 1997;29:1371–1379.

24. Asahara T, Chen D, Tsurumi Y, et al. Accelerated restitution of endothelial integrity and endothelium-dependent function after phVEGF165 gene transfer. Circulation 1996;94:3291–3302.

25. Swanson N, Baron J, Hogrefe K, et al. Novel delivery of vascular endothelial growth factor delivery using polymer-coated stents: loading and elution characteristics. Heart 2000; 83:P28(abstract).

26. Costa MA, Sabaté M, van der Giessen W, et al. Late coronary occlusion after intracoronary brachytherapy. Circulation 1999;100:789–792.

27. Armstrong J, Holt CM, Stratford P, Cumberland DC. Phosphorylcholine stent coating as a method of local drug delivery: preliminary data from an ex vivo model. Heart 1997;77:P47(abstract).

28. Armstrong J, Gunn J, Holt CM, et al. Local angiopeptin delivery from coronary stents in porcine coronary arteries. Eur Heart J 1999;20:1929(abstract).

29. Grube E, Gerkens U, Oesterle E et al. Inhibition of in-stent restenosis by the Quanam Drug Delivery polymer stent, in humans followed for up to 8 months. JACC 2000:34A (abstract).

30. Jordan MA, Tosos RJ, Wilson L. Mechanism of mitotic block and inhibition of cell proliferation by taxol at low concentrations. Proc Natl Acad Sci 1993;90:9552–9556.

31. Sollott SJ, Cheng L, Pauly RR, et al. Taxol inhibits neointimal smooth muscle cell accumulation after angioplasty in the rat. J Clin Invest 1995;95:1869–1876.

32. Keelan PC, Miyauchi K, Caplice NM, et al. Modification of molecular events in coronary restenosis using coated stents: the Mayo Clinic approach. Semin Intervent Cardiol 1998;3:211–215.

INDEX